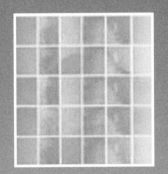

Simulation Simplified

A PRACTICAL HANDBOOK FOR NURSE EDUCATORS

Sandra Goldsworthy, RN, MSc, CNCC, CMSN
Coordinator Critical Care e-Learning Program
Durham College
Assistant Professor
Collaborative BScN Program
Durham College/University of Ontario Institute
 of Technology

Leslie Graham, RN, MN, CNCC
Professor, Nursing
BScN Collaborative Nursing Program
Critical Care e-Learning Certificate Program
Durham College

. Wolters Kluwer | Lippincott Williams & Wilkins
Health
Philadelphia · Baltimore · New York · London
Buenos Aires · Hong Kong · Sydney · Tokyo

Senior Acquisitions Editor: Elizabeth Nieginski
Digital Acquisitions Editor: John Jordan
Product Manager: Eric Van Osten
Design Coordinator: Joan Wendt
Illustration Coordinator: Brett MacNaughton
Manufacturing Coordinator: Karin Duffield
Prepress Vendor: Aptara, Inc.

9 8 7 6 5 4 3 2 1

Printed in the United States of America

Library of Congress Cataloging-in-Publication Data
Goldsworthy, Sandra, 1961–
    Simulation simplified : a practical handbook for nurse educators / Sandra Goldsworthy, Leslie Graham.
      p. ; cm.
    Includes bibliographical references and index.
    ISBN 978-1-4511-4470-3 (alk. paper)
    I. Graham, Leslie, 1956–   II. Title.
    [DNLM: 1. Education, Nursing–methods.   2. Computer Simulation.   3. Patient Simulation. WY 18]
    610.73076–dc23   2012008461

Care has been taken to confirm the accuracy of the information presented and to describe generally accepted practices. However, the authors, editors, and publisher are not responsible for errors or omissions or for any consequences from application of the information in this book and make no warranty, expressed or implied, with respect to the currency, completeness, or accuracy of the contents of the publication. Application of this information in a particular situation remains the professional responsibility of the practitioner; the clinical treatments described and recommended may not be considered absolute and universal recommendations.

The authors, editors, and publisher have exerted every effort to ensure that drug selection and dosage set forth in this text are in accordance with the current recommendations and practice at the time of publication. However, in view of ongoing research, changes in government regulations, and the constant flow of information relating to drug therapy and drug reactions, the reader is urged to check the package insert for each drug for any change in indications and dosage and for added warnings and precautions. This is particularly important when the recommended agent is a new or infrequently employed drug.

Some drugs and medical devices presented in this publication have Food and Drug Administration (FDA) clearance for limited use in restricted research settings. It is the responsibility of the health care provider to ascertain the FDA status of each drug or device planned for use in his or her clinical practice.

To my wonderful husband and children, for without their constant support this project would not have been possible

To all of the critical care nursing students I have had the privilege of mentoring over the years

Sandra Goldsworthy

To my family for their ongoing love and support, always

To my nursing mentors who give so willingly

Leslie Graham

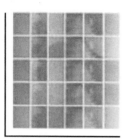

Video Reviewers

Annette Bourgault, PhD(c), MSc, RN, CNCC(C), CNL
Clinical Nurse Leader Program Director, Dept. of Physiological and
    Technological Nursing
Georgia Health Sciences University
Augusta, Georgia, USA

Janet Piper, RegN, MScN, CCRN(c)
Health Sciences Lab Specialist, Simulation Laboratory
Sault College of Applied Arts and Technology
Sault Ste. Marie, ON, Canada

Leland J. Rockstraw, PhD, RN
Associate Clinical Professor of Nursing & Assistant Dean, Simulation,
    Clinical & Technology Learning Operations
Drexel University - College of Nursing & Health Professions
Philadelphia, Pennsylvania, USA

Dr. Colin Torrance RN, DipLScN, BSc(Hon), PhD
Professor in Health Professional Education/Head of Simulation
University of Glamorgan, Glyntaff Campus
Pontypridd, UK

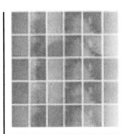

Foreword

*T*eaching students through simulation is rapidly becoming the norm as a method to prepare student nurses prior to actual clinical experience. While simulation has wonderful potential to better prepare students, and protect patients, there exists a lack of material to prepare both the students and instructors.

In this excellent publication, the issue of instructor and student preparation for hands on simulation preparation is met. The authors, some of the best in the world in simulation education, use their extensive experience in simulation to prepare an easy to follow, concise and extremely helpful program for any school using simulation. This text can save the instructor enormous amount of time in preparing for simulation and provide the student with a productive and thorough simulation experience.

In my background in computer simulation, I have been seeking a complimentary approach to transition from the content that can be taught via the computer to content taught in simulation labs. This combined author and student publication is the best transition work I have seen.

The authors have done a wonderful job of developing a publication that will both enrich the student experience and provide an incredibly valuable resource to the faculty in preparing and implementing simulation education. It is exciting to see that faculty have a strong resource to support their use of simulation education. I look forward to using this publication in my teaching and hope you have the same impression as I do.

Thomas Ahrens PhD RN FAAN
Research Scientist
Barnes-Jewish Hospital

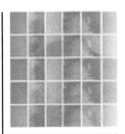

Preface

Welcome to *Simulation Simplified*! This text has been designed for nurse educators/faculty in both academic or practice settings. The aim of this instructor manual is to "simplify" the process of teaching with simulation by providing many helpful tips, scenarios, and templates that you will be able to use right away. The goal of this book is to promote excellence in simulation education.

The lessons learned from this text and accompanying electronic resources will help take the mystery, guess work, and difficulty out of the components of implementing simulation. You will learn how to create realism in your scenario, how to effectively design and unfold a simulation scenario. In addition, you will learn how to facilitate high quality debriefing/reflective thinking sessions after the simulation has been implemented. This text provides a practical approach to delivering effective simulation education to nurses.

An Overview of *Simulation Simplified*:
Simulation Simplified consists of an instructor text, a student handbook, and accompanying electronic resources. The instructor book comprises six chapters. The following is a brief overview of those chapters and the information they contain:

Chapter 1 Introduction
This chapter provides an overview and introduction to simulation in nursing education. Definitions of common terms are presented. Advantages and challenges of implementing simulation education are presented.

Chapter 2 Setting the Stage: Making It Real
In chapter 2, practical strategies for creating realism in simulation cases are presented. Approaches to the simulation setting, equipment needed, faculty preparation, and student preparation are presented.

Chapter 3 The Art of Unfolding the Scenario
In this chapter, a "recipe card" approach is presented. This systematic approach to designing effective simulations will take you through a step-by-step approach to preparing for, implementing and debriefing simulation scenarios. Templates are provided for the instructor to build your own scenarios from start to finish. These templates will save you time in preparation for delivery of simulation education. In addition to the templates, 10 complete ready-to-use cases are provided in this text.

Chapter 4 Debriefing
This chapter provides helpful tips on how to facilitate a debriefing session once the simulation has been completed. Attributes of a successful reflection and debriefing process are presented along with common pitfalls to be avoided.

Chapter 5 Evaluation in Simulation

This chapter provides helpful tips for providing feedback to students during and after simulation exercises. Competency checklists are introduced along with sample templates for evaluation of skills demonstrated during the simulation case.

Chapter 6 International Perspectives on Simulation and Future Directions

In the final chapter, you will gain insight into international perspectives on simulation and future directions projected for the development of simulation education strategies.

Appendices

In the appendices of the *Simulation Simplified* Instructor text, you will find 10 comprehensive simulation scenarios complete with lab results, doctor's orders, pre-tests, and post-tests. In addition, a template for creating your own unique simulation cases is included to help save your valuable teaching preparation time.

Pedagogical Features

Learning Objectives and Chapter Summaries

Each chapter begins with a list of learning objectives that will assist the reader to focus his or her reading. All chapters include a summary and a section outlining chapter key points to highlight the main take home messages.

References

A list of current references cited in the chapter is given at the end of each chapter.

Appendices

The 11 appendices provide 10 complete critical care simulation cases and a template to design new cases and are ready to be used immediately in your own simulation lab.

Glossary

A glossary is found at the end of the book that defines key simulation terms.

Electronic Resources

Electronic instructor resources for *Simulation Simplified* include the following:

- Ten complete video vignette critical care simulation cases. These cases are designed to accompany the 10 cases outlined in the instructor text and the accompanying student handbook.
- An answer key to all student handbook questions with accompanying references.
- Suggested pre-reading for all 10 cases.
- ThePoint. (http://thepoint.lww.com) It is a web-based course and content management system that provides every resource, instructors' and students' need in one easy-to-use site. Advanced technology and superior content combine at thePoint to allow instructors to design and deliver online and offline courses. Students can visit thePoint to access supplemental multimedia resources and enhance their learning experience.
- Access to regularly updated information used for reference in hospital settings: Lippincott's Nursing Advisor and Lippincott's Nursing Procedures and Skills. See the Simulation Simplified access card for more details.

It is with great pleasure we introduce these resources—the instructor textbook, the student handbook and the online package—to you. One of our primary goals in creating these resources has been to promote excellence in critical care nursing simulation practice so that nurses can enhance their skills in a safe environment and ultimately increase the levels of high quality, safe patient care. It is our intent that these resources will provide critical care educators, both in the academic and practice setting, with practical strategies for application in order to deliver effective simulation to aspiring critical care nurses.

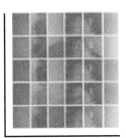

Acknowledgments

We would like to acknowledge Elizabeth Nieginski for her vision, dedication and ongoing support of this project. We would also like to acknowledge the professionalism and dedication of John Jordan, Eric Van Osten and all of the team at LWW in helping make this project a reality.

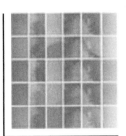

Contents

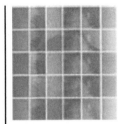

Chapter 1

Introduction

The use of high-fidelity human simulation has exploded into the nursing education context over the last few years and shows no signs of slowing down. Simulation is the replication of the important aspects of a clinical situation in a controlled laboratory setting " . . . so that the situation can be more readily understood and managed when it occurs for real in clinical practice" (Morton, 1995, p. 76). Initially, many simulation labs were created in schools of nursing through widespread funding that became available for adoption of simulation technology and now many labs are being initiated within the hospital and practice setting. The creation of these new simulation labs with high-tech human

simulators has been embraced by many educators, but has left many others with multiple questions and more than a little anxiety on what to do next after the equipment arrives. Maybe you have been in this situation, feeling a little unsure how to begin to implement a simulation program and how you might add this new teaching strategy to your current teaching skill set and practices. We have encountered several educators who report that their simulation equipment is "still in the box" and that beginning simulation programs are overwhelming at times and hard to "know where to start."

▼ GOALS

Our goal is to share some of the lessons we have learned since initiating our simulation program and mentoring many nursing faculty along the way. The resources provided in this text and the accompanying electronic components will provide you with a step-by-step process to implement an engaging teaching–learning environment through the use of high-fidelity human simulation. Mini video vignettes and photos will accompany all chapters and will provide you with a visual resource as you learn the steps to deliver successful simulations. In addition, 10 sample scenarios will be provided in the Appendices A–J with clear instructions on how to develop further scenarios for your lab through our "recipe card" method. Resources that accompany this book are the student handbook and the electronic resources. The student workbook provides accompanying learning exercises, critical thinking questions, and reflective questions that build their knowledge base before and after the simulation. This workbook will help students to prepare for the simulation and will provide follow-up lessons to deepen and augment the learning from the simulation scenario.

Definitions

Before we get started, it is important to define some of the key terms used in simulation. Simulation is the "art and science of recreating a clinical situation in an

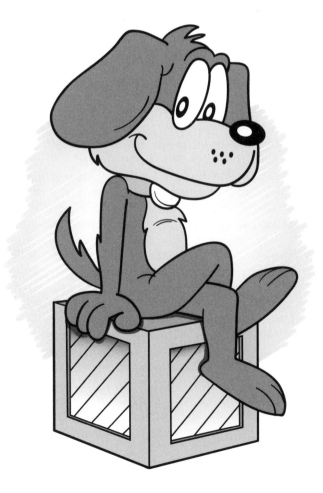

artificial setting..." (G. Gomez & Gomez, 1987) and allows for "deliberate practice in a controlled environment" (Hicks, Coke & Li, 2009). The level of fidelity (or degree of realism) can be described along a continuum (Jeffries, 2007). Fidelity ranges from low fidelity to high fidelity. Some examples of low-fidelity simulation would be injection pads used for practicing injections or an IV cannulation simulation device. Moderate fidelity would include human simulators that do not have chests that rise during breathing or may not have vocal sounds. Finally, a high-fidelity human simulator would have the highest degree of realism, and is typically run via a computerized program, and has a chest that rises and falls with respirations and has vocal sounds.

▼ SIMULATION IN NURSING EDUCATION

Simulation originated primarily in the airline industry where pilots and flight crews practiced in simulated environments in order to prepare them for decision making during critical incidents while in flight (Eaves & Flagg, 2001). Later, simulation was used in anesthesia education to teach step-by-step approaches to psychomotor skills such as intubation (Traver, 1999). In health care, some of the first simulators emerged in the 1960s and included "Resusci-Anne" for resuscitation scenarios and "Harvey" that was used primarily for cardiology training (Cooper & Taqueti, 2004).

High-fidelity human simulation has increasingly emerged on the nursing education front since the early 1990s. However, simulation has been used in nursing education for many years in the form of role playing, practice case scenarios, and low-fidelity applications such as mannequins on which to practice cardiopulmonary resuscitation (CPR). Early versions of low-fidelity simulation were primarily limited to rubber or plastic body parts to practice skills such as catheterization. Today, simulation has evolved to include human-like simulators that can talk, seizure and have a multitude of breath sounds, heart sounds and bowel sounds among other functions. These human high-fidelity simulators are operated through computer-generated programs and can be attached to cardiac monitors showing all related waveforms for analysis such as hemodynamic waveforms (pulmonary artery [PA] catheters, arterial lines, and central lines) and cardiac rhythms. If you have not purchased your equipment for your simulation lab yet, we recommend that you consider the highest fidelity possible within your lab budget. This will allow you the versatility to run a variety of basic medical-surgical scenarios as well as advanced level critical care scenarios.

In today's nursing context, nurse educators are challenged to provide high-quality learning experiences for both nursing students and for practicing nurses to main-tain and learn new skills. Regardless of the intent of the simulation (i.e., remediation, evaluation, orientation), the nurse educator must work within the current hospital or academic setting budget, space, and time constraints. More than ever before, there is a need to have new nurses "up and running" to full productivity as quickly as possible since the reality is that new graduate nurses are being hired into specialty areas (i.e., critical care) that have increasingly high turnover rates. Limited clinical placements for student nurses can pose a challenge for educators trying to ensure optimal learning experiences. Simulation is a teaching strategy that can offer opportunities to provide orientation for new nurses, remediation of lapsed skill sets or for practice of high-risk, low-frequency skills. The simulation lab can also provide educators with a mechanism of both assessing and evaluating skill sets, decision making, and ability to critically think within rapidly changing situations. Furthermore, simulation can provide a strategy to certify employees with specific skill sets (i.e., defibrillation). Teaching and learning with simulation is multi-faceted and can be used to prepare, remediate, or strengthen skill sets among new or experienced nurses.

▼ ADVANTAGES AND CHALLENGES OF SIMULATION

Advantages

Teaching through high-fidelity simulation has many advantages but can also present a few challenges. In preparing nursing graduates for the future, nurse educators must take the current work environment realities into consideration. New graduates as well as experienced nurses are facing increasingly high technology in the practice setting along with the need to critically analyze, prioritize, and make rapid decisions in a complex health care environment. Learning through simulation allows the nurse to be exposed to a variety of controlled clinical situations in which there is the ability to develop skill sets that would otherwise be risky to engage in as a novice with actual patients. Learning through simulation provides a safe, relatively risk-free environment where no harm will come to patients. By practicing in a safe environment, students are able to work within teams and build their confidence as they build their competence (Campbell & Daley, 2009; Jamison, Hovancsek, & Clochesy, 2006; Sears, Goldsworthy, & Goodman, 2010). There are still potential risks in the simulation environment; one example of this would be the use of live defibrillators. Scenarios can be paused and repeated allowing the nurse to build their confidence and competence through practice. A second try in a safe environment shows that improved outcomes are immediately evident (Campbell & Daley, 2009, p. 6).

Every student can be exposed to the same clinical experience through simulation which allows for standardization of assessment and evaluation of progress. In addition, simulation allows the instructor to create situations that may not necessarily occur at any given time within the clinical setting (i.e., cardiac arrests, management of PA catheters). Furthermore, simulation can promote patient safety and high-quality care by teaching vigilance and potentially improving failure to rescue outcomes (Campbell & Daley, 2009). Another advantage of simulation is that the learning becomes student-focused versus teacher-focused allowing the scenario to unfold versus having the instructor take over in an unsafe situation as they would in the actual practice setting. Students receive immediate feedback and are able to engage in critical reflection of their actions, decisions, communication, and skill sets. Through reflective debriefing exercises, the student is able to reformulate a plan and carry out a new plan. Students learn much more than psychomotor skills during the simulation scenarios and are also able to work through emotional and sensitive issues such as a family member who is extremely angry or upset, end-of-life scenarios, or family conferences.

Simulation provides a highly engaging and interactive learning environment for students versus a passive learning experience. Research has shown that when students are highly engaged and actively learning, they have increased retention (Johnson & Zerwic, 1999) and that simulation is more effective than reading or lecture methods. Our experience is that students come early to simulation lab and often want to stay later to practice or have another "run through". Simulation allows for nonlinear thinking versus linear (learning one thing at a time) and allows students to practice with multiple events occurring allowing a better application of theory to practice by identifying connections between concepts (Hicks et al., 2009) (Table 1-1).

Table 1-1. Advantages of Simulation

- Can pause and repeat the scenario
- Safe environment, no harm to patients
- Highly engaging and interactive
- Builds confidence and competence
- Can standardize learning for all students
- Can expose students to situations that may not occur frequently in the clinical setting
- Immediate feedback can be given
- Critically reflective learning enhanced
- Can work through emotional or sensitive situations
- Potential to speed acquisition of skills

Challenges

Although there are many positive aspects of simulation, there are several challenges that must be anticipated and planned for. If you are just beginning your simulation program, you will need to consider the types and numbers of equipment to purchase. Simulators can be very costly ranging from $30,000 to approximately $250,000 per high-fidelity simulator. Initially, try to consider the objective, purposes, and numbers of students that you will be using your simulators for. This will help you to decide what level of fidelity you require. For instance, if you plan on conducting medical-surgical or critical care scenarios, you will likely need to purchase high-fidelity human simulators. Another consideration is ongoing maintenance and upgrading of equipment which can be costly, if not planned for initially.

Space and time may also be a challenge to consider when initiating a simulation program. Do you have a dedicated space to run the scenarios and store any additional equipment (i.e., ventilators, 12-lead machines, intra-aortic balloon pumps, and IV poles)? If simulators are to be left out and set up, this will save time when setting up for a simulation scenario. If they are stored away after each use, you will need to factor in time ahead of the simulation and after for set up and take down. This takes approximately an hour or more depending on the amount of props and equipment to accompany the scenario. This will be explained further in Chapter 2. You may also want to consider space or a dedicated room for the debriefing. Since simulation has become such a popular teaching strategy, simulation lab time may be at a premium, so careful scheduling needs to occur to maximize the resources.

Faculty preparation and workload is also an important component of a successful simulation program since not only do the faculty require specialty nursing experience, they also need to acquire a proficient level of technical computer skill in order to run the simulation. Often when equipment is purchased, there is limited hands-on training provided by the vendors and faculty become overwhelmed and frustrated. A strong initial education session needs to be implemented as well as ongoing investment in professional development for educators as skills develop. We have found that a mentorship program with experienced simulation faculty can be very beneficial in helping build skill in simulation delivery. Human resources may be a challenge since simulation scenarios are typically run with small instructor–student ratios for the best outcome and engagement of students. We recommend an instructor–student ratio of 1:5 for best results. In addition to the human resource needs, time must be allotted for faculty to develop and try scenarios. Developing simulation scenarios is typically more time intensive than preparing lectures (Rauen, 2001). Although there have been several texts published with readymade scenarios, "one size does not fit all" and scenarios must be individualized to your curriculum and learning outcome needs. The fit of the simulation scenario within the teaching–learning context must be examined and not merely "plugged in" but rather carefully integrated so that it makes sense to the learner. Although we will provide you with 10 sample scenarios in this text (see Appendices A–J), we will also provide a template for building your own unique scenarios.

Another challenge when running simulations is to ensure that you create a realistic and believable scenario for the student. The "student's role in simulation needs to be as authentic as possible for transfer of knowledge to occur" (Campbell & Daley, 2009, p. 5). If the student does not believe the simulation is realistic, there is a danger that they may not take it seriously and, therefore, if an error is made they may also not take that seriously as a result. Psychological fidelity has been defined as the degree the participant feels the simulation is realistic and environmental fidelity refers to the realism of the environment (Hicks et al., 2009). We will discuss strategies for creating a realistic and believable environment in Chapter 2 (Table 1-2).

Table 1-2. Challenges of Simulation

- Cost of simulators, supporting equipment
- Ongoing maintenance
- Low instructor-to-student ratio for best outcome
- Faculty preparedness and readiness
- Investment in training of faculty
- Creating a realistic, believable scenario (environmental and psychological fidelity)
- Space and time
- Simulation lab access

▼ SUMMARY

In this chapter, advantages and challenges of implementing a simulation program have been discussed. Simulation has been shown to have many applications among nursing education including preparing new nurses, remediation of lapsed skills, orientation of novice nurses to new practice areas, evaluation, assessment, and recertification. Simulation allows us to sequence learning and provide standardized experiences to all participants. Among some of the most compelling advantages of simulation are its highly interactive nature and its ability to increase confidence and competence among new or experienced nurses while practicing skill sets in a safe environment where no direct harm can occur to patients. Simulation is much more than simply teaching psychomotor skills but rather allows students to work within a team environment and develop skills in critical thinking, clinical reasoning, prioritization, and decision making. Simulation also allows us to teach vigilance and focus on patient safety while also allowing students to work through emotional, ethical, and sensitive issues that are ever present in the clinical landscape. In the following chapters, a practical step-by-step approach will provide you with tips and advice on how to begin to implement your own simulation program successfully.

References

Campbell, S., & Daley, K. (Eds.). (2009). *Simulation scenarios for nurse educators: Making it real.* New York: Springer Publishing.

Cooper, J., & Taqueti, V. (2004). A brief history of the development of mannequin simulators for clinical education and training. *Quality and Safety in Health Care, 13*(Suppl): i11–i18.

Eaves, R., & Flagg, A. (2001). The US Air Force pilot simulated Medical unit: a teaching strategy with multiple applications. *Journal of Nursing Education, 40*, 110–115.

Gomez, G., & Gomez, E. (1987). Learning of psychomotor skills: laboratory versus patient care setting. *Journal of Nursing Education, 26*(1), 20–24.

Hicks, F., Coke, L., & Li, S. (2009). The effect of high fidelity simulation on nursing students knowledge and performance: A pilot study. *National Council of State Boards of Nursing, (NCSBN), 40*, 1–35.

Jamison, R., Hovanscek, M., & Clochessy, J. (2006). A pilot study assessing two methods of teaching intravenous cannulation. *Clinical Simulation in Nursing Education, 2*(1), 1–17.

Jeffries, P. (Ed.). (2007). Simulation in nursing education. National League of Nursing, Laerdal publications.

Johnson, J., & Zerwic, J. (1999). Clinical Simulation Laboratory, an adjunct to clinical teaching, *Nurse Educator, 24*(5), 37–41.

Morton, P. (1995). Creating a laboratory that simulates the critical care learning environment, *Critical Care Nurse, 16*(6), 76–81.

Rauen, C. (2001). Using simulation to teach critical thinking skills. *Critical Care Nursing Clinics of North America, 13*(1), 93–103.

Sears, K., Goldsworthy, S., & Goodman, B. (2010). The relationship between simulation and medication safety. *Journal of Nursing Education, 49*(1), 52–55.

Traver, S. (1999). Anesthesia simulators: concepts and application. *American Journal of Anesthesia, 26*, 393–396.

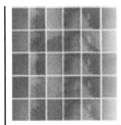

Chapter 2

Setting the Stage: Making It Real

*S*imulation, as a teaching strategy, has been around since nursing students practiced injecting into oranges. Now, through the use of technology, we are able to replicate simple skills to complex case scenarios in order to boost student confidence and competence. When preparing for simulation, you cannot overplan! Much of the work of simulation is done behind the scenes in order to facilitate a seamless learning opportunity. In this chapter you will find the basics for getting the simulation up and running.

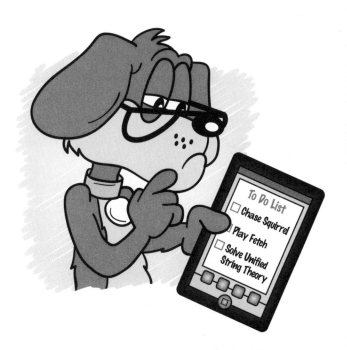

▼ SIMULATION SETTING

First things first—you will need an area to offer the simulation. In designing the simulation lab, establish partnerships with other educators, both clinical and academic. Collaborating with other health professionals, including biomedical departments will bring a wealth of resources for the simulated learning experience. The venue may be as basic as a spare patient room to a more sophisticated learning center and everything in

between. Plan the space to be flexible, yet realistic to mirror the clinical environment. Planning for a separate control room with a two-way mirror will allow the facilitator to have full view of the students. Adding to *authenticity*, as well as to adapt from one unit to the next, the use of professionally made backdrops create the clinical atmosphere. These curtains are ordered as a preplanned unit or can be custom made to replicate your unit. If on a budget, borrow privacy screens, and mount posters to create a realistic hospital environment. Glue color copied pictures to mimic a headboard of the bedside unit.

When booking the space, consider both the area for the simulated patient encounter as well as an area to debrief. An adjacent classroom, a staff lounge, or a small private area equipped with white boards or flip chart paper will work well. As computer technology is also a necessity, have a laptop, LCD, and DVD available to provide limitless educational prospects. Ideally, the ability to videotape or have live streaming will enhance the learning opportunity. At a later date, as faculty become more experienced, complex technologies can be added such as microphones and remotely operated scenarios. Simulation labs are busiest Monday to Friday, necessitating off-hour bookings. Nights and weekends are becoming more popular as simulation experiences are expanding. Wherever you are setting up the simulation experience, be it the hospital auditorium or the university learning centre, space is at a premium, so book rooms well in advance (Figure 2-1).

▼ EQUIPMENT

It is a good idea to review your learning outcomes to identify the simulators and equipment you will need. The use of high-, moderate-, and low fidelity simulators is dependent on the learning outcomes. The use of high-fidelity simulators is using life-like computerized mannequins that mimic real-life situations. The student can listen to their lungs, heart, and bowel sounds while watching the chest rise and fall. The student can listen to the moderate-fidelity simulator's heart, bowel

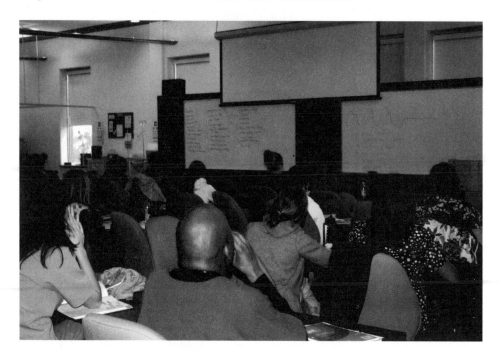

Figure 2.1 Simulation learning environment

and breath sounds, but the chest will not rise and fall. Through the use of the low-fidelity simulator, such as an IV cannulation arm, psychomotor skills can be learned. There are many different types of simulators with a variety of uses (Jefferies, 2007). When securing funding for your simulator, complete a needs assessment to ensure the purchase of a simulator to meet the unique requirements of the hospital or university. Having all the bells and whistles does not ensure that learning occurs. Book the simulator to best meet the needs of your students. The human high-fidelity simulator allows the student to interact with a (almost!) life-like patient that encourages clinical decision making in a safe learning environment. When making a large purchase such as a simulator, do not forget to inquire about faculty training, ongoing vendor support, and importantly, service plans.

Secure the necessary equipment to replicate the clinical environment. This can range from crash carts and defibrillators to candy for simulated pills. Use current technology to support knowledge transfer; old equipment may adversely affect the learning outcomes through *negative knowledge transfer* (Hicks, Coke, & Li, 2009). Even with the latest technology and equipment, there are limitations when projecting real-life situations. Rectify this first by acknowledging the differences between the clinical environment and the simulations, then work that limitation into the case scenario (Simon & Raemer, 2009).

Solicit outdated or unused supplies from the various hospital units. Designate a central repository for the donations—you will be amazed at how quickly the contributions will grow. Many of the disposable supplies can be reused for simulation purposes. Carefully keep outer wraps and boxes to enhance realism in the case scenario. Label the supplies used for simulation to avoid inadvertent patient use as well as acknowledge the donor.

Unleash your imagination to create realistic learning environments. Purchased simulated blood can impart

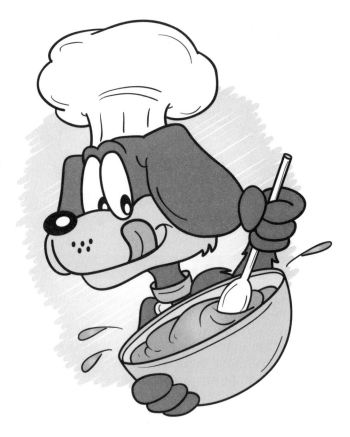

the realism of any trauma brought into the emergency department, mixing red gelatin can form clots, add pudding to a tracheostomy to make sputum, or food colorings with thickeners can reproduce various bodily fluids (Leyk, Harris, & Cleary, 2008). Body sprays can be used to characterize conditions where fruity breath is indicated. Even odors can be purchased in a spray can—not to be confused with air fresheners! Check out your kitchen and start making some interesting concoctions. A word of caution is to try the preparation on a discarded simulator skin to prevent permanent staining of the simulators.

▼ FACULTY

Faculty members play a vital role within simulation. Their ability to coach and mentor the student in a non-threatening manner is foundational to the success of the simulation learning experience. The diverse roles of the faculty are to

- design the curriculum
- develop the learning outcomes
- timing
- sequencing of learning
- unfold the case scenario
- assessing the student's knowledge, skill, and judgment
- facilitate the debriefing
- be sensitive to the learner's emotional well being
- program the simulator
- care for the equipment

Well in advance, select the faculty with the clinical expertise within their specialty. The clinical experts can then respond to a variety of situations depending on student actions. The desired faculty to student ratio is 5:1. It is helpful to have one facilitator unfold the scenario, while another manipulates the simulator. Alternatively, have a simulation technologist familiar with the basic functions of the simulator and the computer programs assist with preprogramming the scenario. All of the faculty should be familiar with basic troubleshooting strategies. Do not forget to enlist the help of others for set up and take down; students or staff may be hired to assist with this part of the simulation. Always have an alternative plan in case of equipment failures—paper-based activities will allow for uninterrupted learning, while affording the faculty time to correct equipment failures.

The next step is to develop learning outcomes or the intent of the simulation. This is often more difficult than it seems. The more the learning outcomes, the longer the simulation. If new to simulation, it is best to stick to 3 or 4 learning outcomes. Learning outcomes should be

- performance related
- contextual
- standard or criterion based
- specific

The scenarios are then developed based on the learning outcomes (Jefferies, 2005). The scenarios at the end of this book can be modified for a particular learning outcome or situation, or develop your own scenarios by using real-life examples from your clinical practice to create rich and meaningful learning experiences. Follow the recipe card to use an easy method of creating your own scenario (see Chapter 3).

In order to deliver this case-based simulation, all faculty should be familiar with the scenario, the equipment, and the simulator. A quick orientation to the computerized program, computer, the simulator and the hook-ups well in advance will help faculty become confident in delivery of the simulation. Do not be intimidated by the number of connections—just follow the step-by-step instruction included by the vendor. This is the opportunity for the faculty to become comfortable with any specialized simulation-related actions such as a hemorrhage or cannulation of the arms. A dry run through is beneficial to iron out any wrinkles before the students arrive.

Unfolding the scenario requires the faculty to be fully in tune with the scenario, the student's practice expectations, and the student actions. This is when the students can be exposed to situations rarely encountered in practice to assist with clinical skill, critical thinking, and clinical judgment. After observing the students enact the simulated clinical case, there is opportunity for the faculty to provide feedback. It is during *debriefing* that expert communication skills are used to guide the students toward reflective practice (Jefferies, 2007).

At the end of the simulation experience, the faculty then asks for student feedback (verbal or written) as well as making note of what would be helpful for future simulation experiences.

▼ STUDENT

The students experience great anxiety related to the unknown of simulation. They may feel inadequate or that their job depends upon successfully completing this simulation. To help build student success, send out pre-learning packages 4 weeks in advance. Students need ample time to do their part in simulation—come prepared. The pre-learning packages include

- well-identified learning objectives
- overview of the simulation
- description of how the simulators work
- clinical scenarios linked with references to review
- evaluation methods

Students should also be reminded to come dressed in uniforms prepared with stethoscopes, clinical resources such as electronic devices or pocket guides.

statistics such as number of simulation sessions offered, number of participants, and cost (faculty, supplies, and mannequin depreciation) will provide accurate information for any of the reports you are required to prepare.

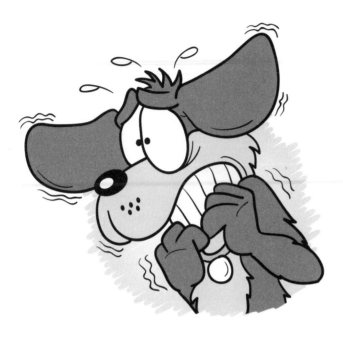

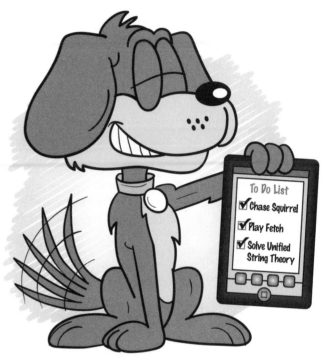

To Do List
☑ Chase Squirrel
☑ Play Fetch
☑ Solve Unified String Theory

▼ READY FOR NEXT TIME!

At the conclusion of each simulation experience, all equipment needs to be stored ready for the next simulation event. Gently washing tape residue and moulage off the simulators will preserve the skin for longer wear. Reservoirs and cannulated arms need to be rinsed and dried before storing. Before storing, according to manufacturer's recommendations, have a signed checklist to indicate all of the smaller pieces are secured with the simulator. Even take photographs to store electronically documenting condition of the returned simulator.

Remember to safely secure all valuable equipment. This can be as simple as well-labeled large clear containers to store equipment based on scenario or similar items. More sophisticated storage systems with wire baskets and high density moveable shelving is also available. Whatever system is used, a checklist of contents will help with inventory control.

It is important to keep meticulous records of any equipment—donated or purchased. This includes serial numbers identifying any warranty and maintenance plans. It is also helpful to keep vendor contact information with a summary of onsite visits as an ongoing reference for future simulation facilitators. Simulation is not done till the paperwork is completed! Keeping the

▼ SUMMARY

In order to maximize the simulated learning experience, it is important to recreate the environment as close as possible to the actual clinical area. Replicate a critical care unit through the use of curtains, portable walls, or screens. Placing equipment commonly found in critical care units such as crash carts or defibrillators enhances the psychological fidelity of the simulation. Review the learning outcomes to match equipment necessary to conduct the simulation. For example, if ECG interpretation is part of the intended learning, have a 12-lead ECG machine with a simulator available. Depending on learning outcomes, select the most appropriate simulator for the scenario. A task trainer may be sufficient for perfecting cannulation techniques, whereas a high-fidelity simulator is required for complex critical care scenarios. When selecting facilitators for the simulation, appoint faculty with relevant clinical expertise. Having experienced faculty will allow a smooth facilitation even with unanticipated events that are common in a simulation. Prepare faculty for the learning environment; orienting to both the scenario and the simulated environment. Thorough student preparation will reduce the anxiety that can often impede learning. Provide students with learning outcomes, an overview of the simulation, describe the function of the simulators, and discuss the evaluation method. By setting the stage and "Making It Real," the student gets to experience the unpredictable clinical setting in a controlled environment.

Box 2-1

Box 2-1. Key Points

- Make the environment as realistic as possible using screens, curtains, posters, or equipment
- Match learning outcomes with appropriate simulator and equipment
- Select faculty with relevant clinical expertise

References

Hicks, F., Coke, L., & Li, S. (2009). The effect of high fidelity simulation on nursing student's knowledge and performance: A pilot study. Vol. 40. *National Council of State Boards of Nursing Research Brief.*

Jefferies, P. (2005). Designing, implementing and evaluating simulations used as teaching strategies in nursing. *Nursing Education Perspectives, 26*(2):96–103.

Jefferies, P. (2007). *Simulation in nursing education from conceptualization to evaluation.* New York: National League for Nursing.

Leyk, M., Harris, K., & Cleary, J. (2008). *Moulage for manikins! or cooking for real dummies.* Willmar, MN: Ridgewater College.

Simon, R., & Raemer, D. (2009). *Debriefing assessment for simulation in healthcare.* Cambridge, MA: Harvard Medical Simulation.

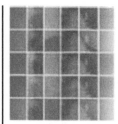

Chapter 3

The Art of Unfolding the Simulation Scenario

*T*o facilitate a successful scenario for maximal student learning, there are a number of critical elements that must be considered. First the scenario must be as realistic as possible. Strategies for creating this level of realism are discussed in Chapter 2. Perhaps one of the most important ways to deliver a successful simulation case is to be prepared with a solid systematic plan. We refer to this as the **"Simulation Recipe Card."** There are three components to the recipe card which include

Part 1: The Overview

Part 2: The Simulation Case

Part 3: The Pre-test and Post-test Questions.

In the following section, each component will be discussed in detail with the goal of providing you a step-by-step approach to unfolding each of your simulation scenarios. In addition to the recipe card, we have provided you with 10 comprehensive scenarios that are ready to use right away in your simulation lab. There is also a blank template provided in order for you to create your own scenarios with our easy-to-use step-by-step system for running a successful simulation.

▼ STEP 1: REVIEW THE OVERVIEW TEMPLATE

How to Use Each Section:

The overview template is a brief synopsis of what will occur in the scenario. The goal of this template is to provide the instructor with a brief overview to the planned simulation (Table 3-1).

Learning Objectives

This resource provides a template for you to plan your scenario from start to finish. It begins with the learning goals. These goals or desired outcomes for learning must be carefully considered before planning the scenario. Common pitfalls at this stage are not carefully planning the intended learning by not having well-defined

Table 3-1. The Overview Template
Learning objectives
Equipment needed
Introduction • Administer pre-test
Body of scenario
Conclusion
Debrief • Administer post-test

outcomes or trying to squeeze too many learning outcomes into a 20-minute scenario. When outcomes are not clearly defined and not reviewed with the students before beginning the scenario, it is very easy to take the case in many different directions and get off course. In the second instance when there are too many learning outcomes, this will become frustrating for both you as the facilitator and the students. To stay on course and maximize the learning opportunity, choose a primary learning outcome with several related goals. See examples in appendices with sample scenarios (Box 3-1).

Box 3-1. Key Tips
• Have well-defined learning outcomes. • Do not create too many learning outcomes for a 20-minute scenario.

Equipment Needed

In this section, all equipment needed for the scenario is listed. It is important to think of everything you will need ahead of time in order to enhance the realism of the case. Once this list is made, it will save you a lot of time in setting up and planning for your scenario. Make sure to include the specific roles on name tags that you would like to include in the scenario.

Introduction

The introduction includes the administration of the pretest questions to the students and the opening or beginning of the scenario. In this section you would include the initial status of the patient (i.e., vital signs, hemodynamic parameters).

Body of Scenario

The body of the scenario describes what will happen with the patient in the case. Typically, this part of the simulation is where the patient becomes unstable or a complication develops.

Conclusion

The conclusion of the scenario is what is expected to happen at the end of the scenario just before the debriefing phase. The conclusion is where you need to get into the scenario within the allotted timeframe.

Debrief

The debriefing period is the timeframe when the posttest questions are administered and the instructor facilitates the post-case debriefing. The essential elements of debriefing will be discussed in the following chapter.

▼ STEP 2: THE CRITICAL CARE SIMULATION

Title of the Case: _____

Scenario number:	**Scenario purpose:**
Scenario focus:	**Learning objectives:**
Scenario level: Critical Care	The student will:
Admission type: ICU	
Patient name:	
Medical record #:	**Learning resources:**
Case number:	Reading assignment:
Date of birth:	**Simulation Student**
Age:	**Workbook activities:**
Gender:	
Attending:	
Scenario start day:	
Scenario start time: 1	
Admitting diagnosis:	
Primary diagnosis:	
Secondary diagnosis:	
Recommended scenario time limit: 20–25 minutes.	
Recommended debriefing time limit: 20–30 minutes.	

RN handoff report

Blood work and doctor's orders (see Appendix X).

Important Components of This Section:

Scenario Focus

The scenario focus is the "working title" for the actual scenario.

Scenario Purpose

The scenario purpose describes the main direction of the scenario.

Patient Information and Learning Preparation Activities

In this section, all of the patient information is listed on the left side of the template, and on the right side, the expected student learning outcomes for the simulation case are listed. In addition, student preparation activities are listed that include reading assignments and student workbook activities. The goal of these activities is to help the student prepare and become more confident in approaching the simulation case. The importance of these activities cannot be stressed enough since this will help decrease the student's anxiety and potentially reduce fear of the unexpected in the simulation.

RN Handoff Report

This area is designed to provide a comprehensive handoff report from one RN to the oncoming RN. All relevant patient history, past and present is provided. The clinical status of the patient will also be presented including current vital signs, cardiac rhythm, IV drip infusions, hemodynamic status, and mechanical ventilation parameters as appropriate. You may decide to present this report in person from one RN to another, by audio or by video.

Doctor's Orders and Lab Results

Doctor's orders and lab values are created for each scenario to enhance the realism of each case. We recommend placing a copy of the doctor's orders, lab values, and an ICU flow sheet on a clipboard at the bedside prior to each scenario. Additional sets of lab values and doctor's orders can be provided to the students in the scenario as the "patient's" condition changes. Blank templates are provided in Appendix K to create your own lab value and doctor's orders (Table 3-2).

How to Use Each Section:

In this section the body of the scenario is unfolded by the facilitator. This part of the simulation incorporates a change in patient status or a complication occurs, a

Table 3-2. Simulation Scenario

Situation/Transition	Facilitator Action	Expected Student Behavioral Outcomes	Resources
Orientation	1. Describe the setting. 2. Describe simulation experience. 3. Review simulator function (if needed). 4. Assign roles and provide name tags.		• Simulator manual

Pre-test (optional)	5. Administer pre-test.
	   a. Online quiz
	      or
	   b. Response system (i.e., i-clickers)
			• Pre-simulation quiz attached
			• I-clicker questions

Report
See instructor script
	6. Provide report by one of the following options:
	   a. Audio
	   b. Video
	   c. Script (instructor read)
	   d. Script (student read)
		1. Student will make notes based on key points of report.	• View RN-to-RN report script
			• I phone download (audio and/or video)
			• video

Start simulation	1. Select scenario ___program file: 2. Start simulation program.		Simulator directions for use manual
Phase I Introduction			
Physiologic state:	3. Progress patient situation following overview recipe card. 4. Select "Phase II Experience" from simulation software menu within 10 minutes. *Recommended time to advance:* 10 minutes		• Overview recipe card #___.
Phase II Body of Scenario			
	5. Progress patient situation following overview recipe card 3.0. 6. Select "Phase II Outcome" from simulation software menu within 10 minutes. *Recommended time to advance:* 5–10 minutes		• Overview recipe card #___.
Phase III Conclusion			
End simulation	7. End scenario. 8. Save debrief log.		• Simulator directions for use manual • Simulator directions for use manual

RN, Registered Nurse.

Table 3-3. Simulation Follow-up

Situation/ Transition	Facilitator Action	Expected Student Behavioral Outcomes	Resources

Debriefing	1. Allow students to discuss experience.
	2. Discuss student performance.
	3. Watch video of simulation (optional).
	4. Administer post-test.
	   a. Online quiz
	   b. Response system
	5. Administer post-simulation survey (optional).
	6. Instruct students to complete self-evaluation/reflection (optional).
	7. Provide remediation, if needed.
		1. Student demonstrates ability to reflect on the scenario and discusses actions that were appropriate and interventions to modify for next time.
		2. Student completes post-test
			• Debriefing/reflection guide
			• Post-simulation quiz
			• Textbook readings:
			• Simulation student workbook activities:

new set of patient information is presented and enough time is allowed for the student to assess and intervene as appropriate. New lab values and doctor's orders are typically presented in this section to accompany the change in status.

Situation/Transition

In this section of the simulation, the new patient status parameters are presented to reflect the complication or rapidly changing status of the patient.

Facilitator Action

The facilitator action section describes what the instructor must do to continue to unfold the scenario. Some examples would include a script that would be relayed to the students or to provide the next set of lab values.

Expected Student/Behavioral Action

Skills and competencies are listed in this area adjacent to the changing status of the patient to describe required student actions. This section can be used to evaluate student performance and/or also as a springboard later in the debriefing section.

Resources

The resource section lists are helpful documents for the facilitator to refer to at various points in the scenario. Initially the overview template is the resource required by the facilitator to orientate to the scenario. Later on in the scenario serial lab values, ECGs, or doctor's orders may be required. In this section, each resource is listed in chronological order as the facilitator would need to access them during the simulation. This prevents the facilitator from having to rapidly search for documents and resources as the case is unfolding.

Concluding the Simulation

Once the transition portion of the simulation has been unfolded, the simulation concludes with another transition in patient status. Examples of the conclusion could include successful resuscitation of a patient or resolution of the complication. The scenario may also end with an unsuccessful resuscitation or end by proceeding to a family conference or by handoff report to the "next shift". If you are repeating the scenario with a different learning group or even the same group, it can be a great learning experience to have the primary nurse provide a handoff report to the "oncoming RN." This will provide an opportunity for the facilitator to assess learning and level of understanding that occurred in the scenario.

Once the scenario has been concluded, the facilitator may move the group immediately into the debriefing session either at the bedside or in a location outside the simulation lab. During the debriefing period, the post-test question can be posed to further enhance and evaluate the learning. In Chapter 4, the debriefing phase will be discussed in detail (Table 3-3).

▼ SUMMARY

In this chapter the key elements of unfolding a successful simulation have been addressed. Important resources for the facilitator have been outlined and a description of each section of the simulation template has been provided. We have provided you with a blank template to create your own scenarios in the appendix of this text as well as online. To help you get started in the delivery of critical care and acute care scenarios, we have also provided you with 10 ready-to-use scenarios in the appendices of this text and in the electronic resources. We recommend that you practice with the templates to become familiar with the content and to make changes or additions to align with your practice context as needed (Box 3-2).

Box 3-2. Key Take-Home Points

- Typical case simulation duration is approximately one hour. Allow 5–10 minutes for orientation to the equipment and setting, 20 minutes to unfold the scenario and 20–30 minutes to debrief the scenario.

- Do not squeeze too many learning outcomes into the scenario. Make it realistic to work through in 20 minutes.

- Review the overview template before beginning the scenario.

- Plan the location and timing of your debriefing session and post-test question delivery.

- Do not lose focus of the objective and goals of the learning for the simulation case.

- Do not hesitate to call a brief "time out" during the scenario if needed to clarify or explain content when knowledge gaps occur.

- Support student learning by providing related reading or activities prior to the case in order to help them prepare and increase their confidence as they enter into the learning.

- Strengthen and extend the learning by assigning follow-up reading and assignments from the student workbook (add title)

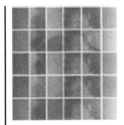

Chapter 4

Debriefing and Providing Feedback: Making Learning Stick

At the conclusion of the simulation scenario, the next phase of learning begins. Debriefing allows the learner to examine the scenario from multiple perspectives in order to achieve a deeper understanding. It is through this detailed analysis that clinical decision making and clinical judgment are developed (Dreifuerst, 2009). In a safe and learner friendly manner, the facilitator expertly engages all of the participants in a reflective journey analyzing skills, behaviors, and attitudes demonstrated during the simulation. The facilitator's role will also include observations from the simulation to enhance communication, prioritization, and teamwork. Through this opportunity to fully examine the simulation, knowledge is developed and learner self-confidence is enhanced.

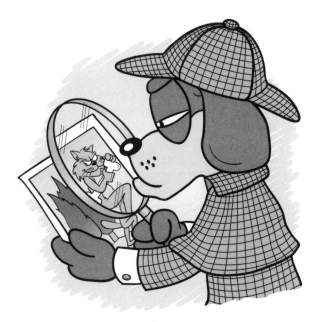

Debriefing, which originated within the military context, occurred after a mission or exercise to fully analyze the event and to develop future plans (Nehring

& Lashley, 2010). Similarly, when debriefing after a nursing simulation, feedback provided can identify tangible measures of improvement when faced with a similar situation. Feedback can also be summative in nature with recommendations for passing a course or being awarded a certificate. Feedback during debriefing should be consistently delivered in a respectful, positive, and encouraging manner (Fanning & Gaba, 2007).

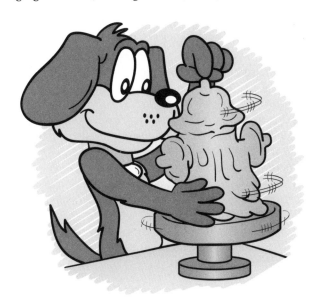

▼ METHODS OF DEBRIEFING

In-Scenario Debriefing

There are several different approaches to debriefing after a simulation. If the learner is struggling during the scenario, the facilitator can "pause" the scenario, to initiate a debriefing (Wickers, 2010). During this form of debriefing, the facilitator can encourage the learner to seek additional resources, that is, cue cards or electronic devices in order to safely proceed with simulation. In promoting student success and boosting confidence, the opportunity to rewind the scenario will be of benefit.

Box 4-1. Recipe Card

Phase III Conclusion of Scenario

Situation/ Transition	Facilitator Action	Student Outcomes
Physiologic state: Patient is not resuscitated	1. Ensures communication with family.	Prepare to go to debriefing session.
Ensures communication occurs with family	2. Debriefing occurs with the health care team.	
Debriefing of health care team		
End Simulation		

Repeating the simulation at a later date can also help the faltering student build their confidence and become successful (Box 4-1).

Small Group Debriefing

At the conclusion of the scenario, the facilitator may wish to debrief right at the bedside. It is a great way to illustrate the learning objectives, especially if these learning objectives include critical care equipment. The facilitator can demonstrate advanced assessment techniques or listen to the simulator's sounds to illustrate the salient points of the scenario. This group of learners can then move into an appropriately sized room, ideally with a round table to discuss the simulation in detail. The facilitator sits within this group, to foster a safe and supportive environment. An alternative to small group debriefing is to facilitate the simulation several times with the small groups then debrief the entire class as a larger group. This method may offer time efficiency with a disadvantage of some learners feeling more inhibited from participating. To enhance the use of simulation as a teaching and learning strategy, the learner can submit a reflection or a journal entry as part of their learning.

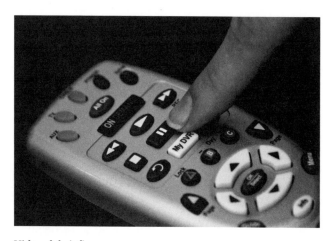

Video debriefing

Video Recorded Debriefing

Video recording of the simulation for playback during the debriefing is another method found to be of benefit. Reviewing the video during the debriefing session encourages the learner to reflect on actual versus imagined performance. It also allows opportunity to review elements the learner may have overlooked during the initial simulation (Fanning & Gaba, 2007; Grant, Moss, Epps, & Watts, 2010). Video recorded simulations are useful for peer feedback to enhance learning. During the simulation, four to five participants are involved in the scenario, while the remainder of the group sits in a media room to view the video. Providing a template or a rubric will also help to focus the learners on the important points of the simulation.

Concept Map Debriefing

To further develop critical thinking and clinical reasoning, the use of concept mapping has been integrated into the simulation (Decker, Moore, Thal, Opton, Caballero, & Beasley, 2010). The learners work in groups using a white board or flip chart paper to create concept maps that are linked to the learning outcomes. Several variations of the same theme can also be beneficial. For example, the learners can work as a group to identify pathophysiology prior to the simulation. After the simulation, the remainder of the concept map can be completed, identifying nursing management. Depending on the learning outcomes, this visual representation contributes to knowledge development and satisfies the varied learning styles.

▼ STEPS TO DEBRIEFING

The debriefing process is considered the most important component of simulation. It is through this deliberate and systematic approach that knowledge, behavior, skills, and attitudes are developed. Debriefing and reflection are teaching–learning strategies that encourage the student to critically analyze their performance to identify gaps and develop a plan of action when faced with a similar situation (Dreifuerst, 2009). First, when debriefing, permit the learner to release any pent-up emotions due to the realism of the scenario. Then as a group, the facilitator identifies the learning outcomes and engages all of the learners to discuss their performance during the simulation in a safe environment. Moving towards a new perspective, the facilitator asks the learners "what will you do differently next time?"

Steps to a Successful Debriefing

Positive Facilitator Attributes

- professional role model
- strong interpersonal skills

- content/subject expertise
- self-awareness and empathy
- acknowledges the diverse background of the learners (Wickers, 2010)
- uses positive coaching and encouragement to promote self-confidence
- assimilates the group into a cohesive team, respectful of each other
- use of silence to encourage self-reflection
- avoid urge to lecture

Box 4-2. Positive Facilitator Approach

Facilitator promotes student success

Active engagement of all participants

Comprehensive examination of simulation

Improve performance

Learning outcomes clearly defined

Insightful and promotes self-discovery

Time out if students falter

Ask probing or cueing questions

Time of debrief ideally same or longer than simulation

Organized, deliberate, and intentional

Reflection on performance

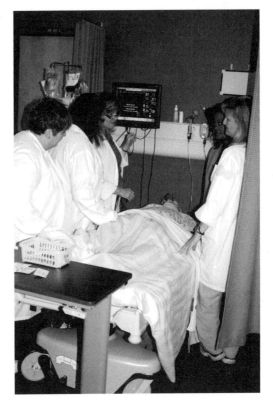

Facilitator debriefing at bedside

Attributes to a Successful Debriefing

- private and appropriately sized space
- a round table, white board, flip chart paper
- viewing screen to review video recorded simulations
- trusting and safe environment
- confidentiality is maintained of simulations and of learner actions
- debriefing should begin as close to the simulation as possible
- length of time allotted for the debriefing should be equal to the length of the simulation to four times the length of the simulation
- allow sufficient time for deep learning and reflection to occur
- facilitator begins the debriefing with restating the learning outcomes, as well as agenda for the debriefing session
- the facilitator in an organized and deliberate manner engages the learner through prompting cues and open-ended questions, that is, "What went well?", "What would you do differently?", "Why did the situation unfold in the manner it did?"

At the end of the debriefing session, the facilitator can summarize the key points. The facilitator can ask the group for final thoughts as way of providing closure to the debriefing. End on a positive note (Simon, Raemer, & Rudolph, 2009).

▼ PITFALLS OF DEBRIEFING

A successful debriefing enhances critical thinking, clinical decision making, and clinical judgment. This requires a facilitator skilled in debriefing techniques. In this role, the facilitator guides the learner towards reflecting on performance in order to gain new knowledge, attitudes, and skills. If debriefing is not conducted in a skillful manner, it can result in psychological harm to the learner. This can occur as a result of a deep emotional link to the fidelity or realism of the simulation. The facilitator needs to be aware of the learner and their composure during the simulation and the debriefing. Further psychological support may be required for those individuals displaying deep emotion such as inconsolable crying. Negative effects may occur for the learner if erroneous learning is not identified and corrected during the debriefing (Dreifuerst, 2009). Without correction, this can lead to unsafe patient situations in the clinical environment. In simulation, the attempt is to mirror the clinical environment, although there are limitations to the simulators and simulation design. This lack of realism can cause anxiety for learners new to the simulation environment. It is important for the facilitator to acknowledge their concerns, redirecting the learner to the learning outcomes. In the debriefing phase, timing is crucial. There will be no benefit gained from the simulation if time is not allotted for the learners to fully debrief. The facilitator must resist answering the questions before the learner has had ample time to provide a thoughtful response. The facilitator debriefing must refrain from focusing entirely on the negative outcomes of the simulation. This tends to undermine the leaner's confidence, as does making the learner feel uncomfortable. The role of the facilitator during the debriefing is significant for optimal learning. The facilitator needs to be aware of their personal style in deliberate and intentional debriefing to promote in-depth learning.

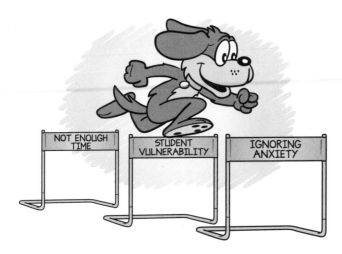

NOT ENOUGH TIME • STUDENT VULNERABILITY • IGNORING ANXIETY

▼ SUMMARY

Debriefing after a simulation enhances the learner's clinical judgment and clinical reasoning abilities. Using a variety of methods, the skilled facilitator guides the learner through reflection to a deeper level of analysis. Equipped with this new learning the challenge for the learner will be to transfer the knowledge and to apply it within the clinical setting (See Box 4-2).

Box 4-3. Key Points

• a skilled facilitator is required for debriefing
• observe learner's reactions to simulation and to debriefing
• correct any erroneous actions in a constructive manner
• acknowledge limitations to simulation
• allot sufficient time to debrief
• avoid rapid fire questions
• allow time for students to answer questions
• avoid totally focusing on negative actions and outcomes
• recognize the vulnerability of the student

References

Decker, S., Moore, A., Thal, W., Opton, L., Caballero, S., & Beasley, M. (2010). Synergistic integration of concept mapping and cause and effect diagramming into simulated experiences. *Clinical Simulation in Nursing, 6*(4), e153–e159.

Dreifuerst, K. (2009). The essentials of debriefing in simulation learning: A concept analysis. *Nursing Education Perspectives, 30*(2), 109–114.

Fanning, R., & Gaba, D. (2007). The role of debriefing in simulation-based learning. *Simulation in Healthcare, 2*(1), 1–7.

Grant, J., Moss, J., Epps, C., & Watts, P. (2010). Using video-facilitated feedback to improve student performance following high-fidelity simulation. *Clinical Simulation in Nursing, 6*(5), e177–e184.

Nehring, W., & Lashley, F. (2010). *High-Fidelity Patient Simulation in Nursing Education.* Sudbury, MA: Jones and Bartlett.

Simon, R., Raemer, D., & Rudolph, J. (2009). *Debriefing Assessment for Simulation in Healthcare – Rater Version.* Cambridge, MA: Center for Medical Simulation.

Wickers, P. (2010). Establishing the climate for a successful debriefing. *Clinical Simulation in Nursing, 6*, e83–e86. doi: 10.1016/j.ecns.2009.06.003.

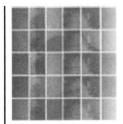

Chapter 5

Evaluation in Simulation

An essential part of teaching with simulation includes evaluating the effectiveness in meeting the learning outcomes. Other components of the simulation session that can be evaluated are the simulation design, student satisfaction, presence of positive educational practices (i.e., positive coaching), and ensuring a standardized approach to the simulation session each time. Through evaluation of these elements, the student's performance will be stronger, simulation-design enhanced and facilitator skills will be further developed (Box 5-1).

Box 5-1. Some Questions to Consider When Evaluating Simulation Experiences

1. Was the experience successful in meeting the learning needs of the students?
2. Were students able to identify problems, potential problems, and changing conditions of the patient?
3. Was the simulation experience at the right level for the experience level of the students? (Was it too difficult or too easy?)
4. Was there enough time to unfold the scenario at a good pace?

▼ SIMULATION EVALUATION TOOLS

The most common type of evaluation that you will likely use in simulation will be checklists to measure skills and competencies. You may also wish to evaluate the effectiveness of the simulation case you have created or assess educational practices at the conclusion of the simulation. Two available tools to assist with the evaluation include the 20-item Simulation Design Scale (SDS, 2005) and the 16-item Educational Practices in Simulation Scale (EPSS, Jeffries, 2007). Each of these tools is completed by the student whereas the skills/competencies checklist is completed by the instructor typically using met or unmet categories. Other tools useful in assessing integration of knowledge from the simulation scenario are the pre-test and the post-test based on the learning outcomes. The student completes the pre-test prior to the simulation case, after completing pre-assigned readings and assignments. The post-test is then administered after the simulation session in order to highlight salient points from the simulation threading concepts such as advanced assessment, integrated data collection, communication skills, and professional comportment.

While it is essential for nurses to develop skills beyond task based, evaluation of complex skills and competencies can be challenging. Simulation is useful in the evaluation of competencies such as clinical judgment based on "knowledge, skilled know-how, and ethical comportment" (Benner, Sutphen, Leonard, & Day, 2010). Depending on simulation design, prioritization and clinical judgment can be assessed using one of the tools presented in this chapter.

Facilitator Feedback

The Lasater Clinical Judgment Rubric (Lasater, 2007) is another tool useful for ensuring consistent evaluation of the students during their performance in simulation. This tool can be used by the facilitator to provide feedback along the way or at the end of the sessions. The student can use the feedback from this tool to document their improvement from one simulation to the next (Lasater, 2007). One of the attributes of the Lasater tool is the use of language that is common to the student, faculty, and the clinical supervisors.

Peer Feedback

Peer critique is valuable in providing feedback to the learner in a non-threatening manner. There are several formats conducive to feedback along the way. To fully support learner success, formative feedback will provide sufficient time for the learner to self-reflect on knowledge, skills, and clinical reasoning. Then, the learner will be provided with an opportunity to demonstrate at a later time mastery of the identified deficiency. Using prompting questions by the facilitator, peer critique can be conducted during the debriefing—either at the bedside or the classroom. Advanced technology such as a video-recorded simulation can be transmitted to peer observers equipped with evaluation templates or rubrics to document observation. In a caring manner, feedback is provided to refocus the learner, promote self-reflection and academic success (Nehring & Lashley, 2010) (Table 5-1).

Table 5-1. Sample Competency Checklists			
Expected Student Actions	**Met**	**Unmet**	**Comments**
1. Student immediately assesses Level of consciousness, ABC			
2. Calls for help and calls a code blue			
3. As soon as the defibrillator arrives, defibrillates at 360 joules after calling all clear twice and looking.			
4. Asks for CPR to be commenced			
5. Physician arrives—asks for the *Dopamine to be run wide open*" student recognizes that this is not safe.			
6. Family member enters room during arrest, very distraught, wants to be at bedside. Student ensures that a team member is present to support family member.			
Feedback:			

▼ SIMULATION: TO PREPARE OR TO EVALUATE STUDENTS?

Should simulation be used solely to help build student's confidence or should it be used to provide a mechanism to test and evaluate skills and competencies? We have found that simulation can be used in both instances. Checklists outlining the important points to be measured or observed can be developed by a panel of content experts, tried and refined. Each competency needs to be separated into individual steps that need to be performed. Checklists are typically completed by the facilitator as the simulation unfolds and individual feedback is provided to the students after the debriefing period. Another method of conducting a final competency assessment or a final exam is to provide the student with a paper-based exam on a clipboard. The facilitator "pauses" the scenario at a predetermined time point and the student answers the question associated with that timeframe in the simulation case. One example of how to use this method is when you are assessing the student's ability to prioritize at a specific timeframe. The facilitator briefly pauses the scenario and asks, for example, the student to list the top three priorities at this point in the scenario. After sufficient time is provided for the student to answer the question, the simulation is resumed.

If simulation is being utilized to prepare students to transition to a new clinical practice area such as the ICU, other evaluation tools such as the General Self Efficacy Tool (GSE) can be used (reference). In general, we have used GSE as a measure prior to simulation (pre-test) and then again after the simulation (post-test). This is helpful in evaluating changes in self-efficacy over time. A Canadian study among undergraduate nursing students measured self-efficacy and medication errors/near misses after a simulation intervention and found that self-efficacy increased in the groups that received the simulation intervention versus the group that did not. There was also less medication errors/near misses in the simulation group compared to the group that did not receive the 24-hour simulation intervention (Sears, Goldsworthy, & Goodman, 2010).

It is important to try or pilot new simulations as you develop them to ensure that the case is meeting the learning needs of the students and it is a robust design that has appropriate timing, is at the right level for the students and the difficulty level is also appropriate for the participants. Having the students evaluate the scenario at the conclusion and reflect over their own learning is important for future evolution and edits to the scenario if needed.

Facilitator Evaluation

One final element of a comprehensive evaluation of the simulation process is evaluation of the facilitator. In response to learner feedback, the facilitator can reflect on personal teaching styles that enhance the learner experience. In developing as a simulation facilitator, several aspects are to be considered:

1. They should be a content expert in the area of the simulation case.
2. They need to be grounded in all aspects of nursing pertaining to that specific simulation. For example, if the learning outcome is to assist nurses to transition to the critical care unit, the facilitator needs to be a critical care nurse and should have experience in the critical care environment. Being a critical care nurse ensures that the scenario design will add to the fidelity of the simulation.
3. They should have expertise in the pedagogy of teaching and learning. In the role of unfolding the scenario

and assessing the students' learning, the facilitator is required to have the ability to deliver the simulation as created to meet the learning outcomes. This may include incorporating real-time situations such as a cardiac rhythm that did not change or vital signs that changed prematurely, into the scenario.

4. They should possess the ability to provide positive coaching skills and encouragement in order to create a safe and positive learning environment. The evaluation of the learner, related to the learning outcomes is sometimes very challenging. There are a variety of learning theories and frameworks that guide this process.

5. They should network with other simulation facilitators to learn new strategies for delivering successful simulations and to promote forward movement of simulation as a science.

▼ SUMMARY

Regardless of the component you are evaluating, it is essential that you are clear about what you want to evaluate and it is also important that the students are clear on what the expectations of the scenario are. If students are unsure of what to expect, it can lead to increased anxiety and tension in the group and can be an impediment to learning through simulation. Before running the simulation, determine the timing of the evaluation; will it be a checklist completed through observation by the facilitator during the scenario, will you "pause" the scenario to evaluate skills such as the ability to prioritize, or will it be a student completed evaluation of the learning experience and the quality of the simulation

experience for their learning. Other evaluations that can be used are self-evaluation (i.e., reflections of learning), peer evaluation, and group versus individual evaluation. Group evaluations can be especially useful in assessing advanced communication skills, team work, and conflict resolution (Box 5-2).

Box 5-2. Key Points

- Clear outcomes and expectations
- Is the evaluation for: Student feedback? Facilitator feedback? Simulation design?
- Use the most appropriate measurement tool for the intended evaluation.
- Deliver all evaluations in a caring, constructive, and positive manner.

References

Benner, P., Sutphen, M. Leonard, V., & Day, L. (2010). *Educating nurses: A call for radical transformation.* San Francisco: Jossey-Bass.

Jeffries, P. (Ed.) (2007). *Simulation in nursing education: From conceptualization to evaluation.* New York: National League of Nursing.

Lasater, K. (2007). Clinical judgement development: Using simulation to create an assessment rubric. *Journal of Nursing Education, 46*(11), 496–503.

Nehring, W., & Lashley, F. (2010). *High-fidelity patient simulation in nursing education.* Sudbury, MA: Jones and Bartlett.

Sears, K., Goldsworthy, S., & Goodman, W. (2010). The relationship between simulation and medication safety. *Journal of Nursing Education, 49*(1), 52–55.

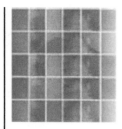

Chapter 6

International Perspectives on Simulation and Future Directions

*S*imulation technology in nursing education has gained momentum and evolved substantially over the last 10 years. Who would have thought that we would be using high-fidelity human simulators in so many innovative ways? Whether preparing nurses for practice or evaluating competencies, one thing is for certain—simulation is here to stay. Early adopters were quick to engage in the use of simulation in nursing curriculum at the undergraduate and the postgraduate level. Some educators who may have been hesitant to "jump on board" have seen the success simulation has had in engaging students and building their confidence in the practice setting. Simulation education is not unique to nursing education in North America and many of our international colleagues have had similar success and challenges in implementing a solid simulation program within the academic or hospital setting. The goal of this chapter is to explore the international perspectives of a number of our nursing colleagues in a variety of countries and to discuss similarities, differences, and innovations in practice. Furthermore, it is the intent of this chapter to present possibilities for future directions in simulation in nursing education. We would like to acknowledge our colleagues from Australia (Professor Michelle Kelly), Wales (Dr. Colin

Torrance), Singapore (Sabrina Koh, Senior Nurse Educator), Greece (Professor Chysoula Lemonidou and Dr. Theodoros Katsoulas), China (Professor Sophia Chan) and Denmark (Professor Jeannette Kirk) for graciously taking the time to be interviewed and sharing the perspective from their respective countries and their insights into the future of simulation education.

▼ STATE OF NURSING SIMULATION

On the international front, the use of simulation in teaching and learning is in a state of flux. From simulation neophyte to the trail blazers, simulation is incorporated into nursing education in varying degrees. In a number of countries, the government has recognized the importance of simulation as a patient safety initiative and provided generous funding. As a result of financial support, these simulation programs are recognized as leaders in the field. Most schools of nursing incorporate simulation in undergraduate education to blend uniquely to and meet the needs of their health care system. In countries such as Singapore well entrenched in the simulation pedagogy, simulation is to a great extent facilitated within the hospital working with postgraduate nurses. Similar to Singapore, Denmark focuses simulation education on the postgraduate nurses.

Simulation has a lot to offer in high-acuity areas such as intensive care units where clinical decision making, clinical judgment, and psychomotor skills need to be performed expediently and accurately. Many countries do not have a credentialed or formal critical care certificate using high-fidelity simulation, however, they do offer advanced scenarios for nurses working in the critical care environment. A number of countries begin critical care education with fourth year undergraduate nurses participating in advanced simulation scenarios using ventilators and hemodynamic monitoring devices. In supporting development of critical care skills, several countries employ a skill station to perfect the psychomotor development and then advance to more comprehensive scenarios. Often critical care is reserved for the more experienced nurse, having advanced preparation at the graduate level.

In order to take simulation to the next level, team training is on the horizon. Many countries engage in interprofessional education (IPE) incorporating simulation. While new to some countries, others have well-established interprofessional simulation offered to a variety of nurses, physicians, and allied health professionals. In Australia, IPE begins in the fourth year, as Dr. Kelly raised the important concept of "role appreciation." Offering IPE to senior students enhanced "role identity" for novice nurses, in addition to exposing medical students to the registered nurses' role. IPE can take many paths from hospital-based to community-based scenarios. In China, IPE is facilitated without the use of simulator. IPE is valued consistently; however, the design is individualized to meet the specific needs.

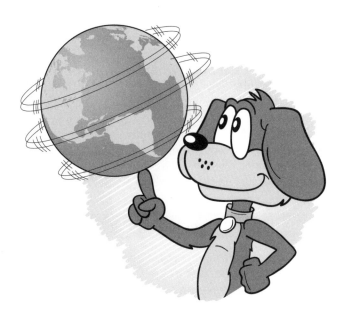

▼ CONTROVERSIES IN SIMULATION

Using simulation as a teaching strategy is a relatively new field that is growing in leaps and bounds. Using this new technology, questions emerged that are not easily answered. As we have come to learn with simulation, "one-size" does not fit all and needs to be tailored to the individual environments. As nurse educators become more comfortable with simulation, traditional teaching–learning strategies are challenged. Through discussion with international partners, themes have illuminated the controversies in simulation.

It was agreed by colleagues in Singapore, Wales, Denmark, and Australia that simulation is becoming increas-

ingly part of nursing education both in the clinical setting and the academic setting. Simulation was identified as an approach to prepare for real-life situations without compromising patient safety. While promoting patient safety and learner confidence, simulation has an important role as a teaching and learning strategy. Professor Kelly added, ". . . while there are early adopters incorporating this technology into nursing education, it takes time for nurse educators to embrace the full use of simulation."

Simulation scenarios developed for areas such as general adult, medical-surgical nursing have been widely accepted, whereas areas such as mental health have slower uptake, especially in UK. Simulation, known to be resource intensive, as such needs to have appropriate funding to fully utilize this technology. In the UK, medical education incorporates a simulation fee for each of their students, whereas nursing education does not incorporate a fee for nursing students. As identified by Singapore colleagues, as a result of a depressed worldwide economy and nursing shortage, there is a subsequent nursing faculty shortage especially, qualified credentialed simulation educators to conduct meaningful simulations. This will have an impact on the use of simulation within nursing education, as well as the advancement of simulation as a teaching and learning strategy. To develop expertise in simulation delivery, three skill sets are critical. The skill sets required to develop ongoing expertise in simulation delivery include content expertise (i.e., critical care), teaching and learning competency (i.e., principles of adult learners), and technology experience and knowledge of simulator function. In addition, we recommend a period of mentoring with experienced simulation instructors in order to develop skill and confidence in successful simulation delivery.

Another area of great debate is the purpose of simulation in teaching and learning. Our colleagues in Singapore and the UK agree that simulation is for coaching purposes only. Emphatically, both professors from Singapore and the UK agreed that simulation is not for summative evaluation or final examination and should not be viewed as punitive. Dr. Torrance commented that the use of simulation is not "sophisticated enough or reliable enough to give each student the same scenario" for evaluation purposes. In Denmark, simulation is used for both summative and formative evaluation. In undergraduate education, a limited form of summative evaluation is necessary in order to proceed to the clinical practicum. In postgraduate education, summative evaluation is predominating, with a focus on knowledge translation. In Canada, we use simulation for both preparing the student and increasing self-confidence, as well as for final evaluation of competencies. In the critical care context, simulation is used almost exclusively for summative evaluation.

▼ FACULTY TRAINING

To fully utilize simulation as a teaching and learning strategy, nurse educator training is required. This method of teaching requires the nurse educator to be competent in many areas such as curriculum development, evaluation, and the technical aspects of using low-, medium-, and high-fidelity simulators. Simulation education and credentialing varies considerably. In the UK, there is a limited selection of simulation courses aimed at faculty education. Dr. Torrance commented that most of the simulation education is learning from experienced simulation faculty, and then taking it to the simulation lab to practice. He predicts that this method of education will change as formal simulation education will be necessary. Similarly, in Australia, staff development is at an early stage. Professor Kelly invites faculty into her simulation classes to provide nursing faculty with the opportunity for an observatory experience using simulation.

As simulation becomes more popular, formal courses are available to provide the required education for simulation faculty. In Singapore, Senior Nurse Educator Koh attended an intense week-long simulation education session in the United States. Subsequently, she has been training other internal faculty. In addition to this role, she is also providing further training for her simulation partners within the same geographic location. Simulation education in Denmark is completed at the Danish Institute for Simulation. This education is divided into two levels, each being three days in duration. A close partnership with the local hospital provides a pool of trained facilitators available to assist with nursing simulation.

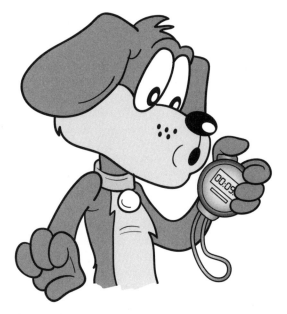

Timing of simulation

▼ TIMING

There was a general consensus among most of the international simulation experts interviewed that effective timing for simulation cases involves delivery of the case over a one-hour period. Specifically, orientation to the equipment, simulation, learning outcomes, and pre-test administration takes place over 10 to 15 minutes. The unfolding of the scenario generally takes place over a 20-minute period with specific learning outcomes and is followed by a 20–30-minute facilitated debriefing session.

▼ DEBRIEFING

The length of debriefing can vary depending on the complexity of the simulation, level of the student, as well as the specific learning outcomes. Debriefing can vary in length, from equal to the time of the simulation or much longer than the simulation. On average, the length of the debriefing was 20 to 30 minutes for a simulation scenario lasting 20 minutes (Figure 6-1).

In order to maximize the learning experience, the instructor-to-student ratio needs to be considered. It was generally agreed among the international simulation experts interviewed that an optimal group size is one instructor to five students. It was also reported that strategies can be utilized for larger groups by having "teams" either observing or actively participating or by using a remote synchronous video that enables the participants not directly involved in the simulation to observe and also participate in the debriefing portion.

▼ METHODS OF DEBRIEFING

Debriefing, considered one of the key elements in simulation is usually held after a simulation to further guide the learner to a deeper analysis of their performance. Furthermore, the concept of multiple ways to debrief after a simulation was validated through the interviews with our international nursing simulation colleagues. When the student has strayed from the intended learning, debriefing was done within the scenario. This temporary pause of the scenario allows the facilitator to guide the students back to the intended learning and simply restart the simulation. As suggested by colleagues in Australia, when facilitating large groups of students, limited time allows for a short debrief at the bedside immediately following the simulation. A longer, more in-depth debriefing takes place at a later date. There is also opportunity to debrief at the bedside, as done in Singapore. The advantage of this method is that the simulator and equipment is in close proximity for further discussion. Debriefing is also facilitated

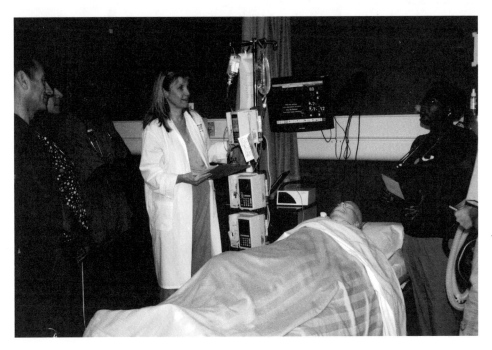

Facilitator debriefing at the bedside

through the use of live video streaming transmitted to the debriefing room, where students critique the performance of the students participating in simulation. To promote trust and protect confidentiality, in Singapore, the video tape used in the simulation is erased in front of the students immediately after the debriefing. In the UK, the simulation is repeated several times until the student achieves maximal learning and mastery of the content. Often, debriefing is conducted in a room where the students can discuss the simulation in depth under the guidance of a skilled facilitator. As Professor Kirk stated "one room is for active engagement, the other room is for (guided) reflection." Through peer and instructor feedback, self-reflection promotes knowledge translation.

▼ WHAT DOES THE FUTURE HOLD? (AKA WHAT ARE THE POSSIBILITIES?)

Unanimously, there was agreement that simulation as a teaching and learning strategy would continue to "gain traction" and grow. While most students like to participate in simulation, it was predicted by Dr Koh that simulation would become mandatory in undergraduate education. She also proposed that, in future, renewal of nursing licensure would include a certain number of mandatory simulation hours. As practicum placements are difficult to secure, especially in specialty areas such as pediatrics and obstetrics, simulation may replace hours in those units. With a nursing shortage looming, Dr. Torrance suggested that simulation is conducive to educating high numbers of nurses. Simulation would

allow for a broader assessment of clinical competencies necessary for practice.

As simulation is a relatively new teaching and learning strategy, faculty need ongoing professional development opportunities to use simulation to its fullest potential. Many of the faculty working in simulation have not had formalized professional development to support the use of this technology. In addition, educators could benefit from sharing international best practices in simulation and begin to develop quality indicators for implementing highly effective simulation practice in teaching and learning.

▼ SUMMARY

From an international perspective, we share the same challenges striving to push the envelope to maximize the full potential that simulation has to offer. In order to ensure the sustainability of simulation, nurse educators need to develop partnerships to share expertise, resources, and ideas. Early adopters can mentor those in the early stages of simulation. As a simulation community, continued research is necessary to provide the evidences to support the use of simulation in nursing education. As a patient safety initiative, simulation will include more simulation promoting interprofessional teams. Through collaboration, sharing challenges and successes, the simulation community can ensure the viability and ongoing successful use of simulation. Globally, one thing was agreed upon: there is no compromise to patient safety. Simulation plays a large role in the education of safe and competent nurses.

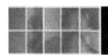

Myocardial Infarction Case 1.0

Overview Recipe Card

Patient Name: Colin Andrew Hawkins

Scenario 1.0

Learning objectives	The student will
	1. Perform a focused assessment based on the patient's complaint or change in patient status.
	2. Recognize normal and abnormal assessment findings.
	3. Prioritize interventions based on findings and assessments.
	4. Document assessment findings.
	5. Perform 12- and 15-lead ECGs.
	6. Demonstrate ability to systematically interpret 12-lead ECG findings.
	7. Demonstrate ability to analyze dysrhythmias and intervene appropriately.
	8. Administer medications accurately and identify indications, contraindications, and side effects associated with interventions.
	9. Call for team assistance as appropriate, which includes initiating a code blue.
	10. Initiate primary ABC measures and safely defibrillate patient needing cardioversion or prepare for cardiac pacing as appropriate.
Equipment needed	12 Lead ECG machine, arterial line setup, peripheral IV line, cardiac monitor, crash cart with defibrillator/pacemaker, nasal cannula O_2 setup, simulated medications, identification band for patient, role name tags for team members, clip board with ICU flow sheet, lab results, 12-lead ECG results and physician's orders, telephone, code blue button.
Introduction	**Administer pre-test.** Sinus rhythm with first-degree block rate of 55, BP 116/55 , RR 20, O_2 saturation 99, Temp 97.7°F (36.5°C)
Body of scenario	Patient progresses from second-degree type 2 heart block (BP drops to 72/42, patient complains of dizziness) to third-degree block to ventricular fibrillation to pulseless electrical activity (PEA).
Conclusion	Patient is not resuscitated. Team plans for communication with family and debriefing with cardiac arrest team.
Debriefing	**Administer post-test.**

Critical Care Simulation

Myocardial Infarction Case 1.0

Scenario number: 1.0
Scenario focus: Myocardial Infarction
Scenario level: Critical Care
Admission type: ICU
Patient name: Colin Andrew Hawkins
Unique number: 1786804
Case number: 1.0
Date of birth: August 12, 1951
Age: 59
Gender: M
Attending: Howard Swan, MD
Scenario start day: Monday
Scenario start time: 1900
Admitting diagnosis: Chest Pain R/O MI
Primary diagnosis: Inferior Myocardial Infarction
Secondary diagnosis: Insulin Dependent Diabetes
Mellitus
Recommended scenario time limit: 20–25
minutes
Recommended debriefing time limit: 20–30
minutes

Scenario purpose: Nursing management of the patient
experiencing myocardial infarction and subsequent cardiac
arrest in a critical care practice setting.

Learning objectives:
The student will
1. Perform a focused assessment based on the patient's
complaint or change in patient status.
2. Recognize normal and abnormal assessment findings.
3. Prioritize interventions based on findings and assessments.
4. Document assessment findings.
5. Perform 12- and 15-lead ECGs.
6. Demonstrate ability to systematically interpret 12-lead ECG
findings.
7. Demonstrate ability to analyze dysrhythmias and intervene
appropriately.
8. Administer medications accurately and identify indications,
contraindications, and side effects associated with
interventions.
9. Call for assistance of team as appropriate including initiating
a code blue.
10. Initiate primary ABC measures and safely defibrillate a
patient needing cardioversion or prepare for cardiac pacing
as appropriate.

Learning resources:
Reading assignment:
1. Morton, P. & Fontaine, D. (2009). Chapter 21. In *Critical Care
Nursing: A Holistic Approach* (9th ed.). Philadelphia:
Lippincott Williams & Wilkins.
2. American Heart Association (2010). 2010 American heart
association guidelines for cardiopulmonary resuscitation and
emergency cardiovascular care. *Circulation*, 122 (Suppl. 3).
S729–S767. DOI: 10.1161/CIRCULATIONAHA.110.970988
3. Sulsa, G., Suffredini, A., McAreavey, D. et al. (2006). *The
handbook of critical care drug therapy* (3rd ed.). Philadelphia:
Lippincott Williams and Wilkins.

Simulation Student Workbook activities:
Myocardial Infarction Case 1.0 in student workbook. Student
to complete pre-simulation.

RN to RN Handoff Report

Colin Hawkins, a 51-year-old Caucasian male patient of Dr. Swan arrived to the ER with chest pain, and an order to rule out
myocardial infarction (MI). He has a history of insulin dependent diabetes and had an anterior/septal MI 12 months ago.
He smokes two packs of cigarettes per day and is approximately 50 pounds over his ideal weight. He was admitted to the
ER complaining of substernal chest pain, "heaviness," and nausea. He was short of breath and diaphoretic on admission.
Medications at home include metoprolol 50 mg daily, atorvastatin (Lipitor) 20 mg, nitroglycerin spray PRN. Currently,
Mr. Hawkins is on oxygen 3 L/min via nasal cannula, IV normal saline solution TKVO in left hand and a saline lock in the
right forearm. He was given the following medications in ER; nitroglycerin spray ×2, aspirin. He is currently not
experiencing chest pain.

He has no known allergies.

He also has a left radial arterial line in situ and Dr. Swan is planning to insert a pulmonary artery catheter shortly.

Current vital signs: Sinus rhythm with a first-degree heart block at 55, B/P 116/55, RR 22, T 98.8°F (37.1°C), O_2 saturation
99% on 3 L/m per nasal cannula.

His blood work results and physician's orders are attached.

Simulation Scenario

Situation/Transition	Facilitator Action	Expected Student Behavioral Outcomes	Resources
Orientation	1. Describe the setting. 2. Describe simulation experience. 3. Review simulator function (if needed).		• Simulator Directions for simulator manual

Pre-test (optional)	4. Administer pre-test.
	   a. Online quiz
	     or
	   b. Response system (i.e., I-clickers)
			• Pre-simulation quiz attached
			 • I-clicker questions

Report (see instructor script)	5. Provide report by one of the following options:
	   a. Audio
	   b. Video
	   c. Script (instructor read)
	   d. Script (student read)
		1. Student will make notes based on key points of report.	• View RN to RN handoff report script
			 • Smart phone download (audio and/or video)
			 • Video

Start simulation	1. Select Scenario ___ program file: 2. Start simulation program. Set up vital signs and beginning of patient parameters.		• Simulator Directions for simulator manual
Phase I Introduction			
Physiologic state: HR 55 bpm (sinus rhythm with first-degree heart block) BP 116/55 mm Hg RR 22 T 37.1 C SaO$_2$ 99% on 3 L/min nasal cannula Right radial arterial line Normal saline at TKVO rate via right peripheral IV line Lab results Troponin level elevated K+ 3.6 Na 137 CBC within normal limits (may add additional values here within normal limits) Rhythm changes to first-degree AV block type II When asked, the patient indicates that they are not experiencing chest pain but feels very dizzy and lightheaded.	3. Progress patient situation following "Overview Recipe Card" Recommended time to advance scenario: 10 minutes	1. Student conducts systematic patient assessment. 2. Student checks orders, lab values, and calculates IV drip rates for accuracy; verbalizes understanding of medications, indications, and side effects parameters to assess. 3. Student assesses all hemodynamic lines, waveforms, and values and demonstrates correct method for zeroing, levelling, and calibrating equipment. 5. Student compares cuff blood pressure to intra-arterial pressure. 6. Student analyzes cardiac rhythm accurately. 7. Student uses advanced communication strategies for communicating with the anxious patient, the patient's family (if present), and other members of the health care team. 8. Student documents accurately on ICU flow sheet.	• Overview Recipe Card 1.0

(Continued)

Situation/Transition	Facilitator Action	Expected Student Behavioral Outcomes	Resources
		10. Student notes second-degree heart block and notifies physician stat, assesses patient vital signs and asks patient if they are experiencing chest discomfort 11. Student asks to see lab work and notes electrolyte levels, BUN and creatinine results, and most recent cardiac markers. 12. Student demonstrates ability to accurately interpret blood work and recognizes abnormal values. 13. Student performs 12- and 15-lead ECG with accurate placement of electrodes and systematically interprets results.	

Phase II Body of Scenario

Situation/Transition	Facilitator Action	Expected Student Behavioral Outcomes	Resources
Physiologic state: Cardiac monitor sounds alarm. Patient progresses into third-degree heart block. Patient complains of being "very lightheaded." BP drops 72/42 mm Hg. Just as transcutaneous pacing is initiated, patient progresses into ventricular fibrillation. Cardiac arrest is called and code blue is initiated. After patient is defibrillated, CPR commences. ACLS guidelines are followed. Patient progresses into PEA. Show idioventricular rhythm. No pulse.	4. Progress patient situation following Overview Recipe Card 1.0. 5. Select "Phase II Outcome" from simulation software menu within 10 minutes. Recommended time to advance scenario: 5 minutes	1. Student demonstrates ability to recognize life-threatening third-degree heart block, need for pacer or inotropes, and calls physician stat. Prepares dopamine infusion using independent double check for dosage calculation. 2. Student notes decreased blood pressure and patient's unstable status and immediately calls for help. When physician arrives, student applies pacer pads, correctly begins to prepare pacemaker initiation watching for capture as the physician adjusts the mA. 3. Upon cardiac arrest, student immediately identifies that defibrillation is the most appropriate emergency treatment. 4. Student begins CPR (high quality compressions and airway management) while defibrillator is prepared. Student ensures high-quality airway management and compressions in between shocks. 5. Student analyzes rhythm (PEA). 6. Student suggests epinephrine 1 mg IV push and CPR as treatment of choice. 7. In collaboration with team, student suggests potential causes for PEA in this circumstance (massive MI).	• Overview Recipe Card 1.0

Phase III Conclusion of Scenario

Situation/Transition	Facilitator Action	Expected Student Behavioral Outcomes	Resources
Physiologic state: Patient is not resuscitated. Student makes sure that communication occurs with family. Debriefing of health care team. End simulation.		1. Student ensures communication with family. 2. Debriefing occurs with the health care team.	Prepare to go to debriefing session.

ER, emergency room; TKVO, to keep vein open; HR, heart rate; RR, respiratory rate; BP, blood pressure; BUN, blood urea nitrogen; SaO$_2$, blood oxygen saturation; CPR, cardiopulmonary resuscitation.

Simulation Follow-up

Situation/Transition	Instructor Action	Expected Student Behavioral Outcomes	Resources

Debriefing	1. Allow students to discuss experience.
	2. Discuss student performance.
	3. Watch video of simulation (optional).
	4. Administer post-test (attached).
	   a. Online quiz
	   b. Response system
	5. Administer post-simulation survey (optional).
	6. Instruct students to complete self-evaluation/reflection (optional).
	7. Provide remediation, if needed.
		1. Student demonstrates ability to reflect on the scenario and discusses actions that were appropriate and interventions to modify for next time.
		2. Student completes post-test.
			• I-clicker questions
			• Post-test
			Simulation Student Workbook follow-up assignment

Lab Results

Patient Identification
Colin Andrew Hawkins
Unique number: 1786804

Test	Result	Normal Ranges
Chemistry Panel:		
Sodium	135	135–142 mEq/L
Chloride	101	98–107 mEq/L
Potassium	4.1	3.5–5.1 mEq/L
Magnesium		1.3–2.1 mEq/L
BUN	7.1	6–20 mg/dL
		(Elderly >60 years old: 8–23 mg/dL)
Creatinine		0.4–1.3 mg/dL
Carbon dioxide, total		22–30 mEq/L
Glucose	70	62–110 mg/dL
Lactate		5–20 mg/dL
Calcium		8.6–10.3 mg/dL
Ionized Calcium		4.8–5.2 mg/dL
Phosphorus		2.4–5.1 mg/dL
HbA1C		4.0–6.7% (of total hemoglobin H)
LDL cholesterol	1.26	<3.4 mmol/L
HDL Cholesterol	4.2	>1.30 mmol/L
Cholesterol	5.80	<5.20 mmol/L
CBC:		
WBC	5.5	$4.5–11.0 \times 10^3$
RBC	5.0	Men: $4.6–6.2 \times 10^6$
		Women: $4.2–5.4 \times 10^6$
Hgb	16.0	Men: 14.0–17.4 g/dL
		Women: 12.0–16.0 g/dL
Hct	48	Men: 42%–52%
		Women: 37%–47%
Platelets	225	$150–300 \times 10^3$

HbA1C, hemoglobin A1c; LDL, low-density lipoprotein; HDL, high-density lipoprotein; CBC, complete blood count; WBC, white blood cells; RBC, red blood cells; Hgb, hemoglobin; Hct, hematocrit.

Test	Result	Normal Ranges
PT	12	12–14 seconds
PTT		18–28 seconds
INR	1.0	0.8–1.2
Liver Enzymes:		
ALT	20	7–56 U/L
ALP	42	38–126 U/L
Amylase	36	30–110 U/L
AST	28	<35 U/L
Cardiac Enzymes		
Troponin I	4.5	<0.03 ng/mL
Serum lactate:		5–20 mg/dL
Arterial Blood Gases:		
Blood pH		7.34–7.44
Bicarbonate		22–26 mEq/L
(HCO$_3$)		
pCO$_2$		35–45 mm Hg
pO$_2$		75–100

PT, prothrombin time; PTT, partial thromboplastin time; INR, international normalized ratio; ALT, alanine transaminase; ALP, alkaline phosphatase; AST, aspartate aminotransferase.

Simulation Hospital

Patient Identification
Colin Andrew Hawkins
Unique number: 1786804
Hospital File

Physician's Order Record

1. Use ballpoint pen.
2. Draw a line through orders not required and initial.

Admitting Diagnosis: Myocardial Infarction Allergies: penicillin	Code Status: Full

Monitoring:
   ✓ Record VS q15min until stable then q1h
   ✓ Continuous cardiac monitoring
   ☐ CVP q1h
   ☐ Pulmonary Artery Occlusive Pressure q1h
   ☐ Cardiac output/cardiac index/SVR q4h	

Activity:
   ✓ Bedrest
   ✓ Position supine with HOB_____degrees
*keep HOB raised greater than 30 degrees when possible	

(Continued)

Diet:
- ☐ NPO
- ✓ Heart Smart
- ☐ 1800 kcal diabetic diet
- ☐ Enteral feedings: Insert small-bore feeding tube and commence feeding.
  Type_____Rate_____
- ✓ Consult dietitian

Other: full fluids
IV:
Total fluid to infuse_____TKVO_____hourly
- ✓ NS TKVO
- ☐ Lactated Ringer's at_____/h
- ☐ D_5W at_____/h
- ☐ Other:_____
- ✓ Hemodynamic lines to maintain patency with NS under pressure

O_2:
Titrate O_2 to maintain SaO_2 greater than 95%
If mechanically ventilated:
ETT inserted by_____at_____cm

Mode:
_____SIMV_____Assist Control_____Pressure Support__Pressure Control_____CPAP
Rate:_____ Tidal volume_____
FiO_2_____ PEEP_____
- ☐ Withhold sedation at 0600 for assessment of weaning

Medications:
- ✓ Aspirin, enteric coated 80 mg PO daily
- ☐ Acetaminophen 650 mg PO q6h PRN pain or temp greater than 38.5° Celsius
- ☐ Ceftazidime 500 mg IV q8h
- ☐ Cefazolin 1g IV q8h
- ☐ Dalteparin 5,000 units SQ daily
- ☐ Furosemide_____mg IV daily
- ☐ Fentanyl_____mcg q1h PRN
- ☐ Heparin 5,000 units SQ q12h
- ☐ Hydromorphone 0.5– 1.0 mg IV q1h PRN
- ☐ Metoprolol_____PO/ng_____
- ☐ Midazolam 2–4 mg IV q1–2h PRN
- ✓ Morphine 2–4 mg IV q1–2h PRN
- ☐ Ondansetron 4 mg q_____h PRN
  Insulin Protocol
capillary blood glucose q2h
Goal 80 to 110 mg/dL
Blood glucose = Units/hour
Less than 70 = off
70–89 = 0.2 unit/hour
90–99 = 0.5 unit/hour
100–129 = 1 unit/hour
130–179 = 1.5 unit/hour
180–239 = 2 unit/hour
240–299 = 3 unit/hour
300–359 = 4 unit/hour

(Continued)

Greater than 20 notify physician
- ☐ Vancomycin_____ g q_____ h IV
- ✓ Other: Enoxaparin 1 mg/kg q12h
- ☐ Voluven_____ mL if urine output less than 0.5 mL/kg/h or CVP less than_____
- ✓ Nitroglycerin 100 mg/250 mL D_5W start at 20 mcg/h to max 200 mcg. Titrate for chest pain.
- ✓ Dopamine 200 mg/250 mL D_5W start at 5 mcg/kg/min. Titrate to maintain systolic B/P greater than 90 mm Hg.
- ☐ Epinephrine 2 mg/250 mL NS at_____ to_____ mcg/min to maintain_____ greater than_____
- ☐ Dobutamine 250 mg/250 mL NS or D_5W at____ to ____ to maintain_____ greater than_____
- ☐ Norepinephrine 4 mg/250 mL D_5W at_____ to_____ maintain_____
- ☐ Vasopressin 20 U/h_____ to_____ to maintain_____ greater than_____
- ☐ Other:

Chest pain protocol:
If chest pain occurs, obtain stat ECG,
- ✓ Nitroglycerin 0.4 mg spray SL PRN for chest pain. May repeat q5min ×2 (maximum 3 doses). Then notify physician.

12-lead ECG on arrival
- ✓ Repeat ECG daily and with chest pain

Lab Tests:
- ☐ Albumin daily
- ☐ Bilirubin daily
- ✓ CBC daily
- ✓ Chemistry daily (electrolytes, glucose, urea, creatinine)
- ✓ Cardiac enzymes and troponin q8h ×3
- ☐ Cross and type_____ units
- ✓ ABG daily and PRN
- ☐ Calcium daily
- ☐ Magnesium daily
- ✓ PTT/PT daily
- ✓ If patient becomes febrile, obtain blood for cultures ×2
- ✓ Sputum for C&S

Diagnostic Tests:
- ✓ Chest x-ray (portable) tomorrow
- ☐ Echo
- ☐ Ultrasound_____
- ☐ CT scan_____

Treatments:
- ☐ Daily weights
- ✓ Delirium score BID
- ☐ Change dressing as per protocol
- ☐ Physio

Other:
Metoprolol 50 mg PO once daily
Lipitor 20 mg once daily

Physician's Signature:_____ Date_____ Time_____
Nurse's Signature:_____ Date_____ Time_____

CVP, central venous pressure; SVR, systemic vascular resistance; HOB, head of bed; NPO, nothing by mouth; TKVO, to keep vein open; NS, normal saline; D_5W, dextrose 5% water; SaO_2, blood oxygen saturation; ETT, endotracheal tube; SIMV, synchronized intermittent mandatory ventilation; CPAP, continuous positive airway pressure; FiO_2, fractional inspired oxygen; PEEP, positive end-expiratory pressure; PO, by mouth; PRN, when necessary; IV, intravenous; SL, sublingually; ABG, arterial blood gas; BID, twice a day.

Pre- and Post-Test Questions

Pre-Test Questions	Expected Answer/Reference
1. Describe the characteristics of the four atrioventricular (AV) blocks.	**Answer: (key characteristics listed, for more detail please see reference below)** **First-Degree AV Block:** prolonged pri >0.20 seconds **Second-Degree AV Block Type 1 (or Wenkebach):** pri gradually lengthens until a beat is dropped and then resets. **Second-Degree AV Block Type 2 (Mobitz 2):** pri is constant with randomly dropped beats, more p waves than QRSs. **Third-degree heart block (Complete Heart Block):** no relationship between p waves and QRSs, more p waves than QRSs. Morton, P., & Fontaine, D. (2009). *Critical Care Nursing: A Holistic Approach* (9th ed., pp. 286–287). Philadelphia: Lippincott Williams & Wilkins.
2. Describe symptoms of a patient experiencing a myocardial infarction.	**Answer:** • Chest discomfort or pain, described often as heaviness, squeezing, or smothering feeling. • The pain can radiate to neck, jaw, shoulders, or back. • Other associated findings include nausea and vomiting, weakness, shortness of breath, pallor, anxiety. Restlessness and diaphoresis. Morton, P., & Fontaine, D. (2009). *Critical Care Nursing: A Holistic Approach* (9th ed., p. 477). Philadelphia: Lippincott Williams & Wilkins.
3. Discuss safety implications during defibrillation.	**Answer:** • Ensure it is a shockable rhythm • Ensure bed is clear and defibrillator operator is clear prior to defibrillation. • Avoid standing in wet areas • Ensure oxygen is removed from bed • Ensure energy level is correct for biphasic or monophasic unit. • Charge paddles on chest • Never carry charged paddles or leave paddles outside of defibrillator. • If using hands-free pads, ensure oxygen pockets are removed and there is good skin contact. ACLS 2010 Guidelines

AV, atrioventricular; ACLS, Advanced Cardiac Life Support.

Post-Test Questions	Expected Answer/Reference
1. Review 2010 ACLS guidelines for treatment of third-degree heart block, PEA, and ventricular fibrillation.	**Answer: (key points, see ACLS guidelines for detail)** **Third-degree AV Block:** In the unstable patient, the treatment required for this rhythm is transcutaneous pacing or a choice of a dopamine infusion at 2–10 mcg/kg/min. or an epinephrine infusion at 2–10 mcg/kg/min. **PEA:** The key treatment for PEA includes high quality CPR, epinephrine 1 mg every 3–5 minutes and a determination and treatment of the potential underlying causes. **Ventricular Fibrillation:** The definitive treatment for ventricular fibrillation is immediate defibrillation, high quality CPR as well as 1 mg epinephrine to be administered after the second defibrillation and 300 mg amiodarone to be administered after the third shock. ACLS 2010 Guidelines
2. Discuss potential causes of PEA	**Answer:** Potential causes of PEA include the following: tension pneumothorax, hypovolemia, hypothermia, hyper/hypokalemia, coronary thrombosis, pulmonary embolus, cardiac tamponade, hypoxia, acidosis, toxins. ACLS 2010 Guidelines
3. If the patient would have been resuscitated, describe post-cardiac arrest care.	**Answer:** **4 key interventions:** 1. Oxygenation and appropriate ventilation (avoid hyperventilation, check endotracheal tube if present, keep oxygen saturation >94, chest x-ray). 2. Fluids and vasoactive care (keep systolic B/P >90, consider reversible causes). 3. Diagnose and treat myocardial ischemia. 4. Therapeutic hypothermia. ACLS 2010 Guidelines
4. Which ECG lead waveforms would you examine to determine an inferior, lateral, posterior, or anterior MI?	**Answer:** **Anterior:** V3 and V4 **Lateral:** I, AVL, V5 and V6. **Inferior:** II, III and AVF **Posterior:** V1 and V2 initially but need to obtain a 15 lead ECG to confirm. Morton, P. & Fontaine, D. (2009). *Critical Care Nursing: A Holistic Approach.* (9th ed., p. 478). Philadelphia: Lippincott Williams & Wilkins.

PEA, pulseless electrical activity; ACLS, Advanced Cardiac Life Support; AV, atrioventricular; CPR, cardiopulmonary resuscitation; MI, myocardial infarction.

Competency Checklist

Myocardial Infarction Case 1.0

Name: **Date:**

Competency	Examples	Met	Unmet	Comments
Performs appropriate assessment.	Focused cardio-respiratory			
12- and 15-lead ECG proficiency.	Performs 12-lead ECG 12-lead ECG Interpretation Performs 15-lead ECG			
Demonstrates ability to correctly interpret arrhythmia	• AV Blocks • Ventricular Fibrillation • PEA			
Demonstrates safe management of hemodynamic monitoring.	Pulmonary artery catheter CVP/PAOP/PCWP Cardiac output Arterial catheter			
Demonstrates safe management of oxygenation.	Ventilation modes Arterial Blood Gas Interpretation Troubleshoots Ventilator alarms			
Demonstrates safe administration of pharmacological agents.	ACLS medications Dopamine or epinephrine infusion			
Accurately interprets lab values.	Chemistry Hematology Troponin Arterial Blood Gases			
Demonstrates ability to quickly recognize and prioritize a patient's rapidly deteriorating condition.	Hypotension Decreased level of consciousness Assessment of chest pain/discomfort			
Demonstrates principles related to safe patient care.	Alarms on Accurate handoff report Communication with patient and health care team Lines secured Independent double checks Positioning			
Specific:	Proper placement of transcutaneous pacemaker pads Follows ACLS algorithm for Ventricular fibrillation, third-degree AV block and PEA Communication with family Initiates code blue High quality CPR			

Feedback: _____

_____

Instructor: _____

PEA, pulseless electrical activity; AV, atrioventricular; CVP, central venous pressure; PAOP, pulmonary artery occlusion pressure; PCWP, pulmonary capillary wedge pressure; ACLS, Advanced Cardiac Life Support; CPR, cardiorespiratory resuscitation.

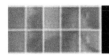

Hypovolemic Shock Case 2.0

Overview Recipe Card

Patient: Elsie Mae Chu

Scenario 2.0

Learning objectives	The student will: 1. Perform a focused assessment based on the patient's complaint or change in the patient's status. 2. Recognize normal and abnormal assessment findings. 3. Prioritize interventions based on findings and assessments. 4. Document assessment findings. 5. Demonstrate principles of safe blood product administration. 6. Recognize signs and symptoms of hypovolemic shock. 7. Discuss potential signs and describe treatment of transfusion reactions in addition to risks associated with multiple transfusions. 8. Demonstrate ability to analyze dysrhythmias and intervene appropriately. 9. Administer medications accurately and identify indications, contraindications, and side effects associated with interventions. 10. Call for team assistance and initiate a code blue as appropriate. 11. Initiate primary ABC measures and safely defibrillate patients needing cardioversion or prepares for cardiac pacing as appropriate.
Equipment needed	12-lead ECG machine, arterial line setup, peripheral IV line, cardiac monitor, crash cart with defibrillator/pacemaker, manual resuscitation device and oral airway, simulated medications, identification band for patient, role name tags for team, clipboard with ICU flow sheet, lab results, 12-lead ECG results and physician's orders, telephone, code blue button, simulated packed red blood cells tubing, IV pumps, normal saline solution, simulated blood and disposable bed pads.
Introduction	Administer pre-test. Cardiac arrest is called in delivery room and ICU nurse responds as part of cardiac arrest team. Patient has ventricular tachycardia with no pulse.
Body of scenario	Patient progresses from ventricular tachycardia with no pulse to sinus tachycardia with frequent PVCs, after one defibrillation, with BP 70/40, RR 24, and shallow breaths. Patient transferred to ICU and mechanical ventilation is initiated. Multiple transfusions of packed red blood cells are administered; patient continues to hemorrhage and has large amounts of vaginal sanguineous drainage.
Conclusion	Patient is stabilized and taken stat to the OR. Family communication ensues and team transfers the patient to OR staff.
Debriefing	Administer post-test.

PVC, premature ventricular contraction; BP, blood pressure; RR, respiratory rate, OR, operating room; ICU, intensive care unit.

Critical Care Simulation

Hypovolemic Shock Case 2.0

Scenario number: 2.0
Scenario focus: Hypovolemic shock
Scenario level: Critical care
Admission type: ICU
Patient name: Elsie Mae Chu
Unique number: 1786805
Case number: 2.0
Date of birth: April 26, 1972
Age: 38
Gender: F
Attending: Priscilla Chambers, MD
Scenario start day: Monday
Scenario start time: 0500
Admitting diagnosis: Pregnancy
Primary diagnosis: Pregnancy
Secondary diagnosis: Intrapartum cardiac
  dysrhythmias
Recommended scenario time limit:
  20–25 minutes
Recommended debriefing time limit:
  20–30 minutes

Scenario purpose: Nursing management of the obstetric patient experiencing hypovolemic shock and subsequent cardiac arrest in a critical care practice setting.

Learning objectives:
The student will
1. Perform a focused assessment based on the patient's complaint or change in the patient's status.
2. Recognize normal and abnormal assessment findings.
3. Prioritize interventions based on findings and assessments.
4. Document assessment findings.
5. Demonstrate principles of safe blood product administration.
6. Recognize signs and symptoms of hypovolemic shock.
7. Discuss potential signs and describe treatment of transfusion reactions in addition to risks associated with multiple transfusions.
8. Demonstrate ability to analyze dysrhythmias and intervene appropriately.
9. Administer medications accurately and identify indications, contraindications, and side effects associated with interventions.
10. Call for assistance of team as appropriate including initiating a code blue.
11. Initiate primary ABC measures and safely defibrillate a patient needing cardioversion or prepare for pacing as appropriate.

Learning resources:
Reading assignment:
1. Morton, P., & Fontaine, D. (2009). *Critical care nursing: A holistic approach.* (9th ed., Chapter 54). Philadelphia: Lippincott Williams & Wilkins.
2. American Heart Association (2010). 2010 American heart Association guidelines for cardiopulmonary resuscitation and emergency cardiovascular care. *Circulation*, 122 (Suppl. 3). S729–S767. DOI: 10.1161/CIRCULATIONAHA.110.97098.
3. Sulsa, G., Suffredini, A., McAreavey, D. et al. (2006). *The handbook of critical care drug therap*y (3rd ed.). Philadelphia: Lippincott Williams and Wilkins.

Simulation Student Workbook activities: Hypovolemic Shock Case 2.0 in student workbook. Student to complete pre-simulation.

RN to RN Handoff Report
Elsie Chu, a 38-year-old Asian female patient of Dr. P. Chambers, is in labor. She is admitted to the Labor and Delivery Unit. Medications at home included maternal vitamins. She states that she drinks 8 cups of ginseng tea per day. On admission, she is pale, anxious, and very weak. She states she is very tired. She has had frequent PVCs during the last 6 weeks of her pregnancy. She has had no previous surgeries but was treated previously for infertility issues. This is her first pregnancy and she has had a weight gain of 25 pounds. Mrs. Chu has IV normal saline TKVO in the left hand and a saline lock in the right forearm.

She has no known allergies.

Blood work results and physician's orders are attached.

About 3 hours later, Mrs. Chu delivers a healthy baby boy, 6 pounds 2 ounces and 20 inches long with Apgar scores of 8 and 10.

Shortly after delivery, Mrs. Chu begins to have large amounts of vaginal, sanguineous drainage. Her blood pressure suddenly drops and she becomes unresponsive. A code blue is called.

PVC, premature ventricular contraction; TKVO, to keep vein open.

Simulation Scenario Introduction

Situation/Transition	Facilitator Action	Expected Student Behavioral Outcomes	Resources
Orientation	1. Describe the setting 2. Describe simulation experience 3. Review simulator function (if needed)		• Simulator Directions for simulator manual

Pre-test (optional)	4. Administer pre-test
	  a. Online quiz
	    or
	  b. Response system (i.e., I-clickers)
			• Pre-simulation quiz attached
			• I-clicker questions

Report (see instructor script)	5. Provide report by one of the following options:
	  a. Audio
	  b. Video
	  c. Script (instructor read)
	  d. Script (student read)
		1. Student will make notes based on key points of report.	• View RN Handover Report script
			• Smart phone download (audio and/or video)
			• Video

Start simulation	1. Select Scenario 2.0 program file: 2. Start simulation program.		• Simulator Directions for simulator manual
Phase I Introduction			
Physiologic state: Cardiac arrest team arrives (includes ICU nurse) Patient in ventricular tachycardia (no pulse) heavy vaginal bleeding	3. Progress patient situation Overview Recipe Card 2.0 4. Select "Phase II Body of Scenario" from simulation software menu within 5 minutes. Recommended time to advance: 5 minutes	1. Student quickly assesses airway, breathing, circulation ABCs), in addition to cardiac rhythm. 2. Student delegates team members to begin CPR, get crash cart, and begin airway management. 3. When defibrillator arrives, student defibrillates patient once, ensuring that all team members are clear by saying "all clear" twice and observing to be sure that team is clear and oxygen is off bed. 4. Student ensures that high-quality CPR is continued after shock.	• Overview Recipe Card 2.0

(Continued)

Situation/Transition	Facilitator Action	Expected Student Behavioral Outcomes	Resources
Phase II Body of Scenario			
Physiologic state: Patient is intubated and manually ventilated with resuscitation bag after one defibrillation Patient's rhythm converts to sinus tachycardia with frequent multifocal premature ventricular contractions BP 70/40 mm Hg Patient not responding to verbal stimuli Patient transferred to ICU Patient continues to have heavy vaginal bleeding. Fundus is impalpable. Two units of packed red blood cells are ordered to be given stat. Normal saline boluses are initiated through two large bore peripheral IVs	5. Progress patient situation following Overview Recipe Card 2.0 6. Select "Phase II Conclusion" from simulation software menu within 10 minutes. *Recommended time to advance:* 5–10 minutes	5. Student assists with intubation and continues to monitor vital signs q5–15 min. 6. Student recognizes that the patient is hypotensive and very unstable, notes heavy vaginal bleeding. Administers normal saline fluid boluses as ordered followed by dopamine infusion titrated to maintain systolic B/P >90 mm Hg ensuring independent double check of dosage calculation with each titration. 7. Student notes change in patient's neurological status. 8. Student checks blood products with another registered nurse and administers appropriately ensuring transfusion reactions are assessed for. 9. Student has another team member update and support patient's husband who is present at the bedside.	• Overview Recipe Card 2.0
Phase III Conclusion			
Physiologic state: Patient is stabilized but still very hypotensive (BP 76/46 mm Hg) Patient continues to bleed heavily and two more units of packed red blood cells are now infusing Physician speaks to husband at bedside and explains that the patient needs to return to the OR to correct cause of bleeding. RN present with physician to support husband at bedside. End simulation	7. End scenario. 8. Save debriefing log.	1. When patient is resuscitated, student assesses blood loss and level of consciousness as well as cardiac rhythm. 2. Continues to assess for potential transfusion reaction. 3. Student attempts to communicate with the patient. 4. Student reassesses vital signs. 5. Student supports husband at bedside and prepares patient for OR.	• Simulator Directions for simulator manual • Simulator Directions for simulator manual

ICU, intensive care unit; CPR, cardiopulmonary resuscitation; BP, blood pressure; OR, operating room.

Simulation Follow-up

Situation/Transition	Instructor Action	Expected Student Behavioral Outcomes	Resources
Debriefing	1. Allow students to discuss experience 2. Discuss student performance 3. Watch video of simulation (optional) 4. Administer post-test 　a. Online quiz 　b. Response system 5. Administer post-simulation survey (optional) 6. Instruct students to complete self-evaluation/reflection (optional) 7. Provide remediation, if needed.	1. Student demonstrates ability to reflect on the scenario and discusses actions that were appropriate and interventions to modify for next time. 2. Student completes post-test.	• Debriefing/reflection guide • Administers post-simulation quiz • I-clicker questions Morton, P. & Fontaine, D. (2009). *Critical care nursing: A holistic approach* (9th ed.). Philadelphia: Lippincott Williams & Wilkins. • Simulation Student Workbook hypovolemic shock follow-up questions.

Lab Results

Patient Identification
Elsie Mae Chu
Unique number: 1786805

Test	Result	Normal Ranges
Chemistry Panel:		
Sodium	135	135–1425 mEq/L
Chloride	101	98–107 mEq/L
Potassium	4.7	3.5 –5.1 mEq/L
Magnesium		1.3–2.1 mEq/L
BUN	7.1	6–20 mg/dL (Elderly >60 years old: 8–23 mg/dL)
Creatinine	80	0.4–1.3 mg/dL
Carbon dioxide, total		22–30 mEq/L
Glucose	70	62–110 mg/dL
Lactate		5–20 mg/dL
Calcium		8.6–10.3 mg/dL
Ionized calcium		4.8–5.2
Phosphorus		2.4–5.1
HbA1C		4.0–6.7% (of total hemoglobin H)
CBC:		
WBC	4.8	$4.5–11.0 \times 10^3$
RBC	3.20	Men: $4.6–6.2 \times 10^6$ Women: $4.2–5.4 \times 10^6$
Hgb	69	Men: 14.0–17.4 g/dL Women: 12.0–16.0 g/dL
Hct	0.58	Men: 42–52% Women: 37–47%
Platelets	200	$150–300 \times 10^3$

BUN, blood urea nitrogen; CBC, complete blood count; WBC, white blood cells; RBC, red blood cells; Hgb, hemoglobin; Hct, hemocrit.

Test	Result	Normal Ranges
PT **PTT** **INR**		12–14 seconds 18–28 seconds 0.8–1.2
Liver Enzymes: ALT ALP Amylase AST Troponin I Serum lactate: Arterial Blood Gases: Blood pH HCO$_3$ pCO$_2$ pO$_2$	10 42 28	7–56 U/L 38–126 U/L 30–110 U/L <35 u/l <0.03 ng/mL 5–20 mg/dL 7.34–7.44 22–26 mEq/L 35–45 mm Hg 75–100 mm HG

ALT, alanine transaminase; ALP, alkaline phosphatase; PT, prothrombin time; PTT, partial thromboplastin time; INR, international normalized ratio.

Patient Identification
Elsie Mae Chu
Unique Patient Number: 1786805

Hospital File

Simulation Hospital

Physician's Order Record

1. Use ballpoint pen
2. Draw a line through orders not required and initial

Admitting diagnosis: Cardiac arrest/hypovolemic shock Allergies: NKDA	Code Status: Full code
Monitoring: ✓ Record VS q15min until stable then q1h ✓ Continuous cardiac monitoring ☐ CVP q1h ☐ Pulmonary capillary wedge pressure q_____h ☐ Cardiac output/Cardiac index/SVR q_____h	
Activity: ✓ Bed rest ✓ Position supine with HOB_____degrees *keep HOB >30 degrees when possible	
Diet: ✓ NPO ☐ Heart smart ☐ 1800 kcal diabetic diet ☐ Enteral feeds: Insert small bore feeding tube and commence feeds. Type_____rate_____ ☐ Consult dietitian Other: Full fluids	

(Continued)

IV:

Total fluid to infuse _____ TKVO_____ hourly

  ✓ NS 0.9% 150 mL/hr

  ☐ Lactated Ringers at _____/hr

  ☐ D_5W at _____/hr

  ✓ Other: Two units packed cells stat then repeat CBC

  ✓ Hemodynamic lines to maintain patency with normal saline under pressure

---

O_2:

Titrate O_2 to maintain SaO_2 >95%

If mechanically ventilated:

ETT inserted by_____ at _____ cm

Mode:

_____ SIMV _____ Assist Control _____ Pressure Support_____ Pressure Control _____ CPAP

Rate: _____ Tidal volume _____

FiO_2_____ PEEP _____

  ☐ Withhold sedation at 0600 for assessment of weaning

Medications:

  ✓ Aspirin enteric coated 80 mg PO daily

  ☐ Acetaminophen 650 mg PO q6h PRN pain or temperature >38.5°C

  ☐ Ceftazidine 500 mg IV q8h

  ☐ Cefazolin 1g IV q8h

  ☐ Dalteparin 5000 units SQ daily

  ☐ Furosemide _____ mg IV daily

  ☐ Fentanyl _____ mcg q1h PRN

  ☐ Heparin 5000 units SQ q12h

  ☐ Hydromorphone 0.5–1.0 mg IV q1h PRN

  ☐ Metoprolol _____ po/ng _____

  ✓ Midazolam 2–4 mg IV q1–2h PRN

  ✓ Morphine 2–4 mg IV q1–2h PRN

  ☐ Ondansetron 4 mg q_____h PRN

  ☐ Insulin Protocol

capillary blood glucose q2h

Goal 80 to 110 mg/dL

Blood glucose = Units/hour

Less than 70 = off

70–89 = 0.2 unit/hour

90–99 = 0.5 unit/hour

100–129 = 1 unit/hour

130–179 = 1.5 unit/hour

180–239 = 2 unit/hour

240–299 = 3 unit/hour

300–359 = 4 unit/hour

20 notify physician

  ☐ Vancomycin_____g q _____h IV

  ✓ Other: Enoxaparin 1 mg/kg q12h

  ☐ Voluven_____mls if urine output <0.5 mL/kg/hour or CVP <_____

  ☐ Nitroglycerin 100 mg/250 mL D_5W start at 20 mcg/hr to max 200 mcg. Titrate for chest pain

  ✓ Dopamine 400 mg/250 mL D_5W start at 5 mcg/kg/min titrate to maintain systolic BP >90.

  ☐ Epinephrine 2 mg/250 mL NS at_____to_____mcg/min to maintain_____>_____

  ☐ Dobutamine 250 mg/250 mL NS or D_5W at_____to_____to maintain_____>_____

  ☐ Norepinephrine 4 mg/250 mL D_5W at_____to_____maintain_____

  ☐ Vasopressin 20 units/hr_____to_____to maintain_____>_____

  ☐ Other:

(Continued)

Chest pain protocol:
If chest pain occurs, obtain stat ECG,
    ☐ Nitroglycerin 0.4 mg spray SL PRN for chest pain. May repeat q5m ×2
        (maximum 3 doses). Then notify the physician

12-lead ECG on arrival   ✓ Repeat ECG daily and with chest pain

Lab tests:
    ☐ Albumin daily
    ☐ Bilirubin daily
    ✓ CBC daily
    ✓ Chemistry daily (electrolytes, glucose, urea, creatinine)
    ✓ Cardiac enzymes and troponin q8h ×3
    ✓ Cross and type 4 units
    ✓ ABG daily and PRN
    ☐ Calcium daily
    ☐ Magnesium daily
    ✓ PTT/PT daily
    ✓ If patient becomes febrile—obtain blood cultures ×2
    ✓ Sputum for C & S

Diagnostic tests:
    ✓ Chest x-ray (portable) now and in am
    ☐ Echo
    ☐ Ultrasound_____
    ☐ CT scan_____

Treatments:
    ☐ Daily weights
    ✓ Delirium score BID
    ☐ Change dressing as per protocol
    ☐ Physiotherapy

Other:
Physician's Signature: _____ Date_____ Time_____ Nurse's Signature: _____ Date_____ Time_____

Pre- and Post-Test Questions

Pre-Test Questions	Expected Answer/Reference
1. Describe safety considerations when double-checking blood products with another registered nurse.	Answer: • Visually check blood unit for clots, unusual color or any leaks. • Check expiry date of unit. • Always check blood unit with another RN at the patient's bedside (unique patient number, blood type and product, ABO and Rh, patient's full name and patient number to be checked to blood unit and name band in the presence of two RNs) • Ensure that there is a signed consent on the patient's chart to receive blood products. • Ensure that doctor's order is present on the chart. • Start blood transfusion without delay after all checks are done. Lima, A. (2010). *Bloody easy: a handbook for health professionals,* Ontario Regional Blood Coordinating Network, Toronto, Ontario. (p. 14 and 16). Retrieved from: http://www.transfusionontario.org/media/HOPE-EN-BloodAdminHdbk-Sprds.pdf Strickler, J. (2010). Traumatic Hypovolemic Shock: halt the downward spiral. *Nursing, 40*(10):34–39; quiz 39–40.

Pre-Test Questions	Expected Answer/Reference
2. Describe symptoms of a patient experiencing hypovolemic shock.	Answer: Tachycardia, hypotension, decreased urine output, thready peripheral pulses, cool clammy skin, tachypnea, decreased level of consciousness. Morton, P., & Fontaine, D. (2009). *Critical care nursing: A holistic approach* (9th ed., pp. 1382–1385). Philadelphia: Lippincott Williams & Wilkins.
3. Which lab values would you assess for in the hemorrhaging patient?	Answer: Decreased hemoglobin, increased serum lactate, changes in hematocrit, electrolyte alterations. Fischbach, F., & Dunning, M. (2009). *A manual of laboratory and diagnostic tests* (8th ed.). Philadelphia: Lippincott Williams & Wilkins.

Post-Test Questions	Expected Answer/Reference
1. Describe signs and symptoms of a transfusion reaction.	**Answer:** Watch for 1. Fever, chills, or rigors. 2. Urticaria and other allergic symptoms (hives, swelling, itchiness) 3. Dyspnea or wheezing 4. Hypotension/hypertension 5. Hemolysis, hemoglobinuria 6. Pain (headache, IV site, lumbar, chest) 7. Nausea and vomiting. Morton, P., & Fontaine, D. (2009). *Critical Care Nursing: A Holistic Approach* (9th ed., p. 1296). Philadelphia: Lippincott Williams & Wilkins. Lima, A. (2010). *Bloody easy: a handbook for health professionals,* Ontario Regional Blood Coordinating Network, Toronto, Ontario. (p. 22). Retrieved from: http://www.transfusionontario.org/media/HOPE-EN-BloodAdminHdbk-Sprds.pdf
2. How would you treat a transfusion reaction?	**Answer:** 1. Stop transfusion immediately 2. Maintain IV access but do not flush blood tubing 3. Check vital signs 4. Verify that the patient ID matches the blood lab label 5. Ensure that the blood unit matches the blood lab label 6. Notify the physician but stay with the patient 7. Notify the blood lab as per hospital policy 8. Treat symptoms as ordered by physician Lima, A. (2010). *Bloody easy: a handbook for health professionals,* Ontario Regional Blood Coordinating Network, Toronto, Ontario. Retrieved from: http://www.transfusionontario.org/media/HOPE-EN-BloodAdminHdbk-Sprds.pdf
3. Describe the 2010 ACLS guideline for resuscitation of a pregnant patient.	**Answer:** Key interventions include • Treat as per ACLS algorithms • Do not delay defibrillation • Give typical ACLS drugs • Perform left uterine displacement to relieve aortocaval compression • If no return of circulation by 4 minutes of resuscitative efforts, obstetric and neonatal teams need to consider performing an immediate C-section • Compressions should be performed slightly higher on the sternum • Consider placing patient on a 30-degree angle with a firm wedge support if left uterine displacement by hand is not effective. ACLS 2010 Guidelines
4. What are the risks of multiple transfusions?	**Answer:** Hypothermia, coagulation issues, acidosis. Strickler, J. (2010). Traumatic hypovolemic shock: Halt the downward spiral. *Nursing, 40*(10):34–39; quiz 39–40.

Competency Checklist

Hypovolemic Shock Case 2.0

Name: **Date:**

Competency	Examples	Met	Unmet	Comments
Performs appropriate assessment	Emergency Comprehensive			
12- and 15-lead ECG proficiency	Performs 12-lead ECG 12-lead ECG interpretation Performs 15-lead ECG			
Demonstrates ability to correctly interpret arrhythmia	• Ventricular tachycardia • Sinus tachycardia with PVCs			
Demonstrates safe management of hemodynamic monitoring.	Pulmonary artery catheter CVP/PAOP/PCWP Cardiac output Arterial catheter			
Demonstrates safe management of oxygenation	Ventilation modes Arterial blood gas interpretation Troubleshoots ventilator alarms			
Demonstrates safe administration of pharmacological agents.	ACLS medications Dopamine infusion			
Accurately interprets lab values.	Chemistry Hematology Troponin Arterial blood gases			
Demonstrates ability to quickly recognize and prioritize a patient's rapidly deteriorating condition.	Hypotension Decreased level of consciousness Assessment of chest pain/discomfort			
Demonstrates principles related to safe patient care.	Alarms on Safe defibrillation Accurate handoff report Communication with patient and health care team Lines secured Independent double checks Positioning			
Specific:	Safe blood product administration and assessment for transfusion reactions. Assesses for hemorrhage and related signs and symptoms. Follows ACLS algorithm for ventricular tachycardia Communication with family Initiates code blue High-quality CPR			

Feedback: _____
_____
_____
_____

Instructor: _____

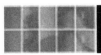

Appendix C

Abdominal Aortic Aneurysm Repair Case 3.0

Overview Recipe Card

Patient: Laura Lewis

Scenario 3.0

Learning objectives	**The student will**
	1. Perform a focused assessment based on the patient's complaint or change in the patient's status.
	2. Recognize normal and abnormal assessment findings.
	3. Prioritize interventions based on findings and assessments.
	4. Document assessment findings.
	5. Analyze and interpret an arterial and pulmonary artery waveform. Perform hemodynamic monitoring, such as right atrial pressure, pulmonary wedge pressure, and cardiac output.
	6. Identify postoperative complications, such as limb ischemia.
	7. Demonstrate ability to analyze dysrhythmias and intervene appropriately.
	8. Administer medications accurately and identify indications, contraindications, and side effects associated with interventions.
	9. Initiate primary ABC measures, administering volume replacements as indicated, managing postoperative pain, troubleshooting ventilator.
	10. Describe nursing management of a surgical patient in the immediate postoperative phase.
Equipment needed	12-lead ECG machine, arterial pressure line and pulmonary artery pressure line, cardiac monitor, crash cart with defibrillator/pacemaker, ventilator, manual resuscitation device, oral airway, disposable gloves, chest tube and chest drainage system/dressing, simulated medications, 1000 mL normal saline solution, IV cannula, IV pole, abdominal dressing, foley catheter with urometer, identification band for patient, role name tags for team members, clip board with ICU flow sheet, lab results, 12-lead ECG results, physician's orders, telephone, and code blue button.
Introduction	Administer pre-test
	HR 100 (atrial fibrillation), BP (cuff) 140/80, (arterial line) 145/70, O_2 saturation 99%, temperature 95°F (35°C), urine output 10 mL
	PAP 28/15, Wedge 9, CVP 5, CI 3.0, CO 4.5, SVR 2200, PVR 250
	Right radial arterial line, right internal jugular, PA line
	Ventilated on SIMV, rate 12, FiO_2 0.50, PEEP 5 cm
	Medications: Propofol 25 mcg/kg/min via side port of introducer, normal saline solution 10 mL/h via side port
	Lactated Ringer's solution 100 mL/h via left peripheral IV line
Body of scenario	Patient begins to emerge from anesthesia, BP increases quickly, HR increases with PVCs, high pressure ventilator alarm, and unable to palpate distal pulses.
	Patient given propofol 25 mcg/kg/min via side port of introducer, normal saline solution 10mL/h via side port, nitroglycerin 30 mcg/min, lactated Ringer's solution 100 mL/h via left peripheral IV line

(Continued)

Conclusion	Arterial line BP 120/70, HR 110 (atrial fibrillation), temperature 97.9°F (36.5°C)
	O$_2$ saturation 98%
	Pulmonary artery occlusive pressure (aka pulmonary artery wedge pressure) 10,
	  CVP 6, CI 3.2, CO 5.0, SVR 1500, PVR 250
	Unable to palpate distal pulses
	Propofol 25 mcg/kg/min via side port of introducer, normal saline solution 10 mL/h
	  via side port, nitroglycerin 30 mcg/min, lactated Ringer's solution 100 mL/h via left
	  peripheral IV line

Debriefing	**Administer post-test**

HR, heart rate; BP, blood pressure; CVP, central venous pressure; CI, cardiac index; CO, cardiac output; SVR, systemic vascular resistance; PVR, peripheral vascular resistance; SIMV, synchronized intermittent mandatory ventilation; PEEP, positive end-expiratory pressure; PVC, premature ventricular contractions.

Critical Care Simulation

Abdominal Aortic Aneurysm Repair Case 3.0

Scenario number: 3.0
Scenario focus: Immediate postoperative care of an abdominal aneurysm repair
Scenario level: Critical care
Admission type: ICU
Patient name: Laura Lewis
Unique number: 1786806
Case number: 3.0
Date of birth: March 9, 1941
Age: 69
Gender: F
Attending: Janice Boyd, MD
Scenario start day: Monday
Scenario start time: 1900
Admitting diagnosis:
  Abdominal Aortic Aneurysm
Primary diagnosis: Abdominal Aortic Aneurysm Repair
Secondary diagnosis:
  Hypertension, pack per day smoker
Recommended scenario time limit: 20–25 minutes
Recommended debriefing time limit: 20–30 minutes

Scenario purpose: Immediate postoperative nursing management of a critical care patient experiencing an abdominal aortic aneurysm repair requiring strict BP control.

Learning objectives:
The student will
1. Perform a focused assessment based on the patient's complaint or change in patient status.
2. Recognize normal and abnormal assessment findings.
3. Prioritize interventions based on findings and assessments.
4. Document assessment findings.
5. Analyze and interpret an arterial and pulmonary artery waveform. Monitor hemodynamic parameters, such as right atrial pressure, pulmonary artery occlusive pressure, and cardiac output.
6. Identify postoperative complications such as limb ischemia.
7. Demonstrate ability to analyze dysrhythmias and intervene appropriately.
8. Administer medications accurately and can identify indications, contraindications and side effects associated with interventions.
9. Initiate primary ABC survey, administering volume replacement as indicated, managing postoperative pain, and troubleshooting ventilator.
10. Describes nursing management of a surgical patient in the immediate postoperative phase.

Learning resources:
Reading assignment:
American Heart Association (2010). 2010 Guidelines for Cardiopulmonary Resuscitation and Emergency Cardiovascular Care. *Circulation*, 122 (Suppl. 3).
Bickley, L., & Szilagyi, P. (2009). *Bates' Guide to Physical Examination and History Taking* (10th ed., Chapter 12). Philadelphia: Lippincott Williams & Wilkins.
Diehl, T. (Ed) (2011). *ECG Interpretation made incredibly easy* (5th ed., Chapter 5). Philadelphia: Lippincott Williams & Wilkins.
Karch, A. (2011). *Lippincott's Nursing Drug Guide*. Philadelphia: Lippincott Williams & Wilkins.
Morton, P., & Fontaine, D. (2010). *Critical Care Nursing: A Holistic Approach* (9th ed., Chapters 13, 17, 19). Philadelphia: Lippincott Williams & Wilkins.
Simulation Student Workbook activities: Abdominal Aortic Aneurysm Repair Case 3.0 in the student workbook. Student to complete pre-simulation.

(Continued)

RN to RN Handoff Report

Laura Lewis is a 69-year-old female patient of Dr. Boyd. She was admitted from the OR with an abdominal aortic aneurysm repair. She has a history of hypertension and is a pack per day cigarette smoker. She was admitted to the ER with complaints of a sudden, "tearing" back pain radiating to her back and hips, associated with nausea and vomiting. She was short of breath and hypotensive on admission. Her initial BP was 90/60 mm Hg in her right arm, 80/55 mm Hg in her left arm, peripheral pulses were weak and thread bilaterally. A pulsatile mass was noted, and on auscultation a bruit was heard. She was immediately taken for an abdominal CT, which revealed a large abdominal aortic aneurysm. Medications at home include aspirin 81 mg, atorvastatin 20 mg, and amlodipine 5 mg BID.

Mrs. Lewis was prepped and taken to the OR for an infrarenal abdominal aortic aneurysm repair with a Dacron graft. At the beginning of the operation, the aorta was noted to be calcified. She was given a general anesthetic as well as propofol throughout the procedure. Her estimated blood loss was approximately 400 mL and she was given 1 unit of packed red blood cells. Vitals signs have remained in the range of BP 90–120/60 mm Hg, sinus rhythm 80–100 bpm. She has a right radial arterial line, a right internal jugular pulmonary artery catheter, propofol infusion at 25 mcg/kg/min via the side port, as well as a no. 18 peripheral IV access via left antecubital fossa. Urine output was 450 mL throughout her time in the OR; her abdominal dressing is dry and intact. As mentioned, Mrs. Lewis is hypertensive and a pack per day smoker. She is being admitted to the ICU for BP control, and ventilatory support. Her husband and daughter are in ICU waiting room.

She has no known allergies.

Blood work results and physician's orders.

OR, operating room; BP, blood pressure.

Simulation Scenario

Situation/Transition	Facilitator Action	Expected Student Behavioral Outcomes	Resources
Orientation	1. Describe the setting 2. Describe simulation experience 3. Review simulator function (if needed)		• Simulator Directions for simulator manual

Pre-test (optional)	4. Administer pre-test
	  a. Online quiz
	  b. Response system (i.e., I-clickers)
			• Pre-simulation quiz attached
			• I-clicker questions

Report (see instructor script)	5. Provide report by one of the following options:
	  a. Audio
	  b. Video
	  c. Script (instructor read)
	  d. Script (student read)
		1. Student will make notes based on key points of report.	• View RN to RN handoff report script
			• Smart phone download (audio and/or video)
			• Video

Start simulation	1. Select Scenario 3.0 AAA Repair program file 2. Start simulation program		• Simulator Directions for simulator manual

(Continued)

Situation/Transition	Facilitator Action	Expected Student Behavioral Outcomes	Resources
Phase I Introduction			
Physiologic state: HR 100 bpm (atrial fibrillation) BP (cuff) 140/80 (arterial line) 145/70 mm Hg SaO$_2$ 99% Temperature 95°F (35°C) Urine output 10 mL straw color urine PAP 28/15 mm Hg PAOP 9 mm Hg CVP 5 mm Hg CI 3.0 L/min/m^2 CO 4.5 L/min SVR 2200 dynes PVR 250 dynes Right radial arterial line Right internal jugular PA catheter Ventilated on SIMV, rate 12, FiO$_2$ 0.50, Vt 500 PEEP 5 cm IV/Infusions: i) Propofol 25 mcg/kg/min via side port of introducer/cordis ii) NS 10 mL/hr via side port iii) Ringer's lactate 100 mL/hr via left peripheral IV	3. Progress patient situation following Overview Recipe Card 3.0 4. Select "Phase II Experience" from simulation software menu within 10 minutes. *Recommended time to advance:* 10 minutes	1. Student receives report, checks orders, lab values and conducts systematic patient assessment. 2. Student checks and calculates IV infusion rates for accuracy; verbalizes understanding of medications, indications, side effects, and important parameters to assess. 3. Student assesses all hemodynamic lines, waveforms, values, and demonstrates correct method for zeroing, leveling, and calibrating equipment. 4. Student demonstrates correct method for obtaining hemodynamic parameters: CVP, wedging PA catheter and performing cardiac outputs. 5. Student compares cuff BP to arterial BP. 6. Analyzes cardiac rhythm accurately. 7. Uses advanced communication strategies for communicating with the ventilated patient, the patient's family, and other members of the health care team. 8. Student documents ventilator settings and demonstrates ability to troubleshoot a high-pressure alarm. 9. Demonstrates ability to titrate vasoactive infusions to maintain BP parameters. 10. Notes low urine output. 11. Asks to see postoperative lab work notes CBC, electrolytes, BUN and creatinine, blood sugar, INR, PTT, and most recent ABGs. 12. Demonstrates ability to accurately interpret ABGs. 13. Demonstrates ability to accurately interpret 12-lead ECG.	• Overview Recipe Card 3.0

(Continued)

Situation/Transition	Facilitator Action	Expected Student Behavioral Outcomes	Resources
Phase II Body of Scenario			
Physiologic state: Arterial line BP 190/70 mm Hg HR 130 bpm (atrial fibrillation with PVCs) SaO$_2$ drops to 93% Temperature 95°F (35°C) PAP 45/18 mm Hg PAOP 12 mm Hg CVP 5 mm Hg CI 2.8 L/min/m^2 CO 4.2 L/min SVR 1800 dynes PVR 250 dynes Absent pedal pulses Ventilator alarms: High pressure	5. Progress patient situation following Overview Recipe Card 3.0 6. Select "Phase II Outcome" from simulation software menu within 10 minutes. Recommended time to advance: 10 minutes	1. Student recognizes that the patient is emerging from anesthesia. 2. Student notes elevated BP. 3. Assesses LOC, airway, breathing. 4. Immediately commences nitroglycerin infusion in response to elevated BP. 5. Administers analgesia safely and accurately, based on assessment findings. 6. Initiates active rewarming with warm blankets or external warming device. 7. Performs and interprets hemodynamic parameters accurately. 8. Notes absent pedal pulses. 9. Assesses ventilator alarms and troubleshoots high-pressure alarm. 10. Assesses patient sedation and increases patient sedation appropriately.	• Overview Recipe Card 3.0
Phase III Conclusion			
Physiologic state: Patient is stabilized in the postoperative period: HR 110 bpm (atrial fibrillation) Arterial line BP 120/70 mm Hg Temperature 98°F (36.5°C) SaO$_2$ 98% PAP 30/15 mm Hg PAOP 10 mm Hg CVP 6 mm Hg CVP 6 mm Hg CO 5.0 L/m CI 3.2 L/min/m^2 Absent pedal pulses End simulation	7. Progress patient situation following Overview Recipe card 3.0 8. Select "Phase II Experience" from simulation software menu within 10 minutes. *Recommended time to advance:* 5 minutes 9. End scenario. 10. Save debriefing log.	1. Assesses patient's LOC, airway, breathing and circulation, dressing, peripheral pulses 2. Identifies the abnormalities in the lab results. 3. Attempts to communicate with patient. Updates the family. 4. Reassesses hemodynamic parameters by performing right atrial pressure 5. Verbalizes the need to use a Doppler ultrasound device to assess pedal pulses.	• Simulator Directions for simulator manual • Simulator Directions for simulator manual

HR, heart rate; BP, blood pressure; SaO$_2$, arterial oxygen saturation; PAP, pulmonary artery pressure; PAOP, pulmonary artery occlusive pressure (formerly pulmonary artery wedge pressure); CVP, central venous pressure; CI, cardiac index; CO, cardiac output; CBC, complete blood count; BUN, blood urea nitrogen; ABG, arterial blood gas; SVR, systemic vascular resistance; PVR, peripheral vascular resistance.

Simulation Follow-up

Situation/Transition	Instructor Action	Expected Student Behavioral Outcomes	Resources

Debriefing	1. Allow students to discuss experience
	2. Encourage student to reflect on performance
	3. Watch video of simulation (optional)
	4. Administer post-test
	  a. Online quiz
	  b. Response system
	5. Administer post-simulation survey (optional)
	6. Instruct students to complete self-evaluation/reflection (optional)
	7. Provide remediation, if needed.
		1. Student demonstrates ability to reflect on the scenario and discusses actions that were appropriate and interventions to modify for next time.
		2. Student completes post-test.
			• Debriefing/Reflection guide
			• Post-simulation quiz
			• Textbook
			• Bates Assessment resource/videos
			• Simulation Student Workbook

Lab Results

Patient Identification
Laura Lewis
Unique number: 1786806

Test	Result	Normal Ranges
Chemistry Panel:		
Sodium	135	135–1425 mEq/L
Chloride	106	98–107 mEq/L
Potassium	4.3	3.5–5.1 mEq/L
Magnesium	1.3	1.3–2.1 mEq/L
BUN	7	6–20 mg/dL
		(Elderly >60 years old: 8–23 mg/dL)
Creatinine	1.4	0.4–1.3 mg/dL
Carbon dioxide, total	22	22–30 mEq/L
Glucose	115	62–110 mg/dL
Lactate		5–20 mg/dL
Calcium	8	8.6–10.3 mg/dL
Ionized calcium		4.8–5.2 mg/dL
Phosphorus		2.4–5.1 mg/dL
HbA1C		4.0–6.7% (of total hemoglobin H)
BNP		<100 pg/mL (or <100 ng/L)
CBC:		
WBC	16	$4.5–11.0 \times 10^3$
RBC	4.1	Men: $4.6–6.2 \times 10^6$
		Women: $4.2–5.4 \times 10^6$
Hgb	10.2	Men: 14.0–17.4 g/dL
		Women: 12.0–16.0 g/dL
Hct	36	Men: 42–52%
		Women: 37–47%
Platelets	100	$150–300 \times 10^3$

BUN, blood urea nitrogen; CBC, complete blood count; WBC, white blood cells; RBC, red blood cells; Hgb, hemoglobin.

Test	Result	Normal Ranges
PT **PTT** **INR**	21 1.75	12–14 seconds 18–28 seconds 0.8–1.2
Liver Enzymes: ALT ALP Amylase Troponin I Serum lactate: Arterial Blood Gases: Blood pH HCO_3 pCO_2 pO_2	 0.02 7.33 18 45 165	7–56 U/L 38–126 U/L 30–110 U/L <0.03 ng/mL 5–20 mg/dL 7.34–7.44 22–26 mEq/L 35–45 mm Hg 75–100 mm Hg

ALT, alanine transaminase; ALP, alkaline phosphatase; PT, prothrombin time; PTT, partial thromboplastin time; INR, international normalized ratio.

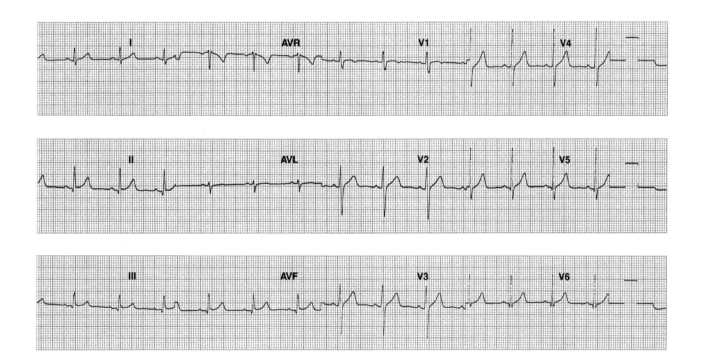

Hospital File

Simulation Hospital

Physician's Order Record

Laura Lewis
Unique Patient Number: 1786806

1. Use ballpoint pen.
2. Draw a line through orders not required and initial.

<table>
<tr>
<td colspan="2">Admitting diagnosis: Abdominal aortic aneurysm repair
Allergies: None
Weight: 70 kg</td>
<td>Code status:
Full</td>
</tr>
<tr>
<td colspan="3">Monitoring:
  ✓ Record VS q15min until stable then q1h
  ✓ Continuous cardiac monitoring
  ✓ CVP q1h
  ✓ Pulmonary capillary occlusive pressure q4h
  ✓ Cardiac output/cardiac index/SVR q4h</td>
</tr>
<tr>
<td colspan="3">Activity:
  ✓ Bed rest *reverse Trendelenburg 30 degrees, may dangle legs at bedside
     tomorrow, mobilize starting tomorrow afternoon
  ☐ Position supine with HOB _____ degrees
*keep HOB raised more than 30 degrees when possible</td>
</tr>
<tr>
<td colspan="3">Diet:
  ☐ NPO until bowel sounds are present then sips
  ☐ Heart smart
  ☐ 1800 kcal diabetic diet
  ✓ Enteral feedings: Insert small-bore feeding tube and commence feeding.
Type TraumaCal
Rate 25 mL progress to 50 mL/hour
  ☐ Consult dietitian</td>
</tr>
<tr>
<td colspan="3">IV:
Total fluid to infuse _____ 125 mL _____ hourly
  ✓ NS at __10 mL/h
  ✓ Lactated Ringer's at __ 100__ /hr
  ☐ D_5W at _____ /h
  ☐ Other:_____
  ✓ Hemodynamic lines to maintain patency with NS solution under pressure</td>
</tr>
<tr>
<td colspan="3">O_2:
Titrate O_2 to maintain SaO_2 >94%
If mechanically ventilated:
ETT inserted by__ S. Acker, RRT, _____ at _____ 25 _____ cm</td>
</tr>
<tr>
<td colspan="3">Mode:
  ✓ _____ SIMV _____ Assist Control _____ Pressure Support _____ Pressure
     Control _____ CPAP
Rate:_____12 _____ breaths/min Tidal volume__500__mL
FiO_2__0.5__ PEEP__5 cm __
  ✓ Withhold sedation at 0600 for assessment of weaning
  ✓ Wean with plans to extubate in am</td>
</tr>
</table>

(Continued)

Medications:
- ☐ Aspirin, enteric coated _____ mg PO daily
- ☐ Acetaminophen 650 mg PO q6h PRN pain or temp more than 38.5°C
- ☐ Ceftazidime 500 mg IV q8h
- ✓ Cefazolin 1g IV q8h
- ☐ Dalteparin 5000 units SQ daily
- ☐ Furosemide _____ mg IV daily
- ☐ Fentanyl _____ mcg q1h PRN
- ✓ Heparin 5000 units SQ q12h, start 12 hours postop if no bleeding
- ☐ Hydromorphone 0.5-1.0 mg IV q1h PRN
- ☐ Metoprolol _____ PO/ng _____
- ✓ Midazolam 2-4 mg IV q1-2h PRN
- ✓ Morphine 2 mg_____ IV q30min PRN
- ☐ Ondansetron 4 mg q_____ h PRN
- ☐ Insulin Protocol

capillary blood glucose q2h

Goal 80 to 110 mg/dL

Blood glucose = Units/hour

Less than 70 = off

70–89 = 0.2 unit/hour

90–99 = 0.5 unit/hour

100–129 = 1 unit/hour

130–179 = 1.5 unit/hour

180–239 = 2 unit/hour

240–299 = 3 unit/hour

300–359 = 4 unit/hour

>20 notify physician
- ☐ Vancomycin _____ g q_____ h IV

Infusions:
- ✓ Voluven __250__mL if urine output less than 0.5 mL/kg/hr or CVP less than__8 mm Hg__
- ✓ Nitroglycerin 100 mg/250 mL D₅W at __10__ mcg/min to max__200 mcg/min__. Titrate to maintain systolic BP 120–140 mm Hg
- ✓ Dopamine 200 mg/250 mL D₅W at __3 mcg/kg/min__ to __10 mcg/kg/min____. Titrate to maintain__systolic__BP__ >120–140 mm Hg or MAP >70 mm Hg____
- ☐ Epinephrine 2 mg/250 mL NS at _____to _____ mcg/min to maintain _____ >_____
- ☐ Dobutamine 250 mg/250 mL NS or D₅W at_____ to _____ to maintain _____ >_____
- ☐ Norepinephrine 4 mg/250 mL D₅W at_____to _____maintain _____
- ☐ Vasopressin 20 U/h _____ to _____ to maintain _____ >_____
- ☐ Other:
- ✓ Propofol 100 mg/10 mL 25–50 mcg/kg/min while on ventilator

Chest pain protocol:

If chest pain occurs, obtain stat ECG,
- ✓ Nitroglycerin 0.4 mg spray SL PRN for chest pain. May repeat q5min × 2 (maximum 3 doses). Then notify the physician.

12-lead ECG on arrival
- ✓ Repeat ECG q8h × 2

(Continued)

Lab tests:
- ☐ Albumin daily
- ☐ Bilirubin daily
- ✓ CBC daily
- ✓ Chemistry daily (electrolytes, glucose, urea, creatinine)
- ✓ Cardiac enzymes and troponin q8h × 3
- ✓ Cross and type_____units *keep 2 units on hand × 48 hr
- ✓ ABG daily and PRN
- ☐ Calcium daily
- ☐ Magnesium daily
- ✓ PTT/PT daily
- ✓ If patient becomes febrile, obtain blood for culture × 2

Diagnostic tests:
- ✓ Chest x-ray (portable) daily
- ☐ Echo
- ☐ Ultrasound_____
- ☐ CT scan_____

Treatments:
- ☐ Daily weights
- ✓ Delirium score BID
- ✓ Change dressing as per protocol
- ✓ Physiotherapy

Other:
- ✓ Maintain systolic BP 120–140 mm Hg, diastolic BP 60–80 mm Hg, MAP 70–100
- ✓ Assess all pulses q1h, notify surgeon if pulse deficit

Physician's Signature:_____Date_____Time_____
Nurse's Signature:_____Date_____Time_____

Pre- and Post-test Questions

Pre-test Questions	Expected Answer/Reference
1. What are the signs and symptoms of an abdominal aortic aneurysm?	• Abdominal or back pain which may be described as "tearing" • Physical examination for the presence of a pulsatile mass and when auscultating bruits are heard • Hypertension (or hypotension) • Blood pressure difference of >10 mm Hg in each arm • Diminished distal pulses Morton, P., & Fontaine, D. (2009). *Critical Care Nursing: A Holistic Approach* (9th ed., pp. 431–432). Philadelphia: Lippincott Williams & Wilkins.
2. Why is tight BP control so important in the postoperative period for a patient undergoing an aortic abdominal aneurysm repair?	• Puts stress or pressure on the fresh suture line, with risk of bleeding • Potential to induce arrhythmias Morton, P., & Fontaine, D. (2009). *Critical Care Nursing: A Holistic Approach* (9th ed., pp. 178–179). Philadelphia: Lippincott Williams & Wilkins.
3. What are the nursing priorities in the immediate postoperative phase for a patient undergoing an aortic abdominal aneurysm repair?	• Monitor airway and breathing every 15 minutes and PRN • Monitor cardiac rhythm continuously; blood pressure and heart rate every 15 minutes and PRN • Maintain normothermia • Monitor urine output • Assess level of consciousness every 15 minutes • Assess pain and comfort • Assess for signs of diminished arterial perfusion Diehl, T. (2012). *Critical Care Made Incredibly Easy* (3rd ed., pp. 260–263). Philadelphia: Lippincott Williams & Wilkins.

Post-test Questions	Expected Answer /Reference
1. What are the complications of an abdominal aortic aneurysm repair?	• Hypoxemia • Hypoventilation • Hypotension • Hypertension • Cardiac dysrhythmias • Hypothermia • Postoperative pain • Nausea and vomiting • Hemorrhage • Spinal cord ischemia • Bowel ischemia Morton, P., & Fontaine, D. (2009). *Critical Care Nursing: A Holistic Approach* (9th ed., p. 175). Philadelphia: Lippincott Williams & Wilkins.
2. Describe DIC.	• DIC is a condition where widespread clotting and hemorrhage occurs • A trigger such as major trauma, shock, sepsis, malignancy, obstetric conditions, intravascular prosthetic devices, prolonged low cardiac output states (shock, prolong cardiopulmonary bypass), surgery, immunological conditions (transplant, blood transfusion reaction), causes the normal coagulation system to be over stimulated • Widespread thrombosis occurs causing depletion of clotting factors and platelets • Simultaneous activation of fibrinolytic system occurs • Signs and symptoms include end-organ ischemia, bleeding into tissues, oozing from intravenous sites, incision sites, gastrointestinal tract, petechiae, hematoma formation • Tests include platelets, fibrin degradation products, prothrombin time, partial thromboplastin time, elevated urea, creatinine • Treatment: monitor vital signs, assess for signs of hemorrhage, assess for evidence of ischemia, trend lab results, identify triggering event, replace clotting factors such as fresh frozen plasma, platelet transfusion, cryoprecipitate, red cell transfusion, minimize venipuncture, apply pressure for at least 15 minutes Morton, P., & Fontaine, D. (2009). *Critical Care Nursing: A Holistic Approach* (9th ed., pp. 1303–1308). Philadelphia: Lippincott Williams & Wilkins.
3. What are the six signs of arterial occlusion?	• Pain • Pulselessness • Pallor • Paresthesia • Paralysis • Poikilothermy Morton, P., & Fontaine, D. (2009). *Critical Care Nursing: A Holistic Approach* (9th ed., p. 429). Philadelphia: Lippincott Williams & Wilkins.

DIC, disseminated intravascular coagulation.

Competency Checklist

Abdominal Aortic Aneurysm Repair Case 3.0

Name: **Date:**

Competency	Examples	Met	Unmet	Comments
Performs appropriate assessment.	Comprehensive Doppler assessment of pulses			
Demonstrates ability to correctly interpret arrhythmia and 12-lead ECG.	Atrial fibrillation			
Demonstrates safe management of hemodynamic monitoring.	Pulmonary catheter CVP/PAOP/PCWP Cardiac output Arterial line			
Demonstrates safe management of oxygenation.	Ventilation modes Endotracheal tube			
Demonstrates safe administration of pharmacological agents.	Propofol Morphine Nitroglycerin Dopamine			
Accurately interprets lab values.	Chemistry Hematology Troponin Arterial blood gases			
Demonstrates ability to quickly recognize and prioritize a patient's rapidly deteriorating condition.	Hypertension Hypotension			
Demonstrates principles related to safe patient care.	Alarms Lines secured Independent double checks Positioning Communication/report			
Specific:	Initiates rewarming postop Communication with health care team/family			

Feedback: _____
_____
_____
_____
_____
_____

Instructor: _____

Closed Head Injury Case 4.0

Overview Recipe Card

Patient: Martin Neylander

Scenario 4.0

Learning objectives	**The student will** 1. Perform a focused assessment based on the patient's complaint or change in the patient's status. 2. Recognize normal and abnormal assessment findings. 3. Prioritize interventions based on findings and assessments. 4. Document assessment findings. 5. Perform 12-lead ECG. 6. Demonstrate nursing management of a patient experiencing a closed head injury. 7. Demonstrate ability to analyze dysrhythmias and intervene appropriately. 8. Administer medications accurately and identify indications, contraindications, and side effects associated with interventions. 9. Initiate primary ABC survey, identifying key priorities to decrease intracranial pressure.
Equipment needed	12-lead ECG machine, pressure arterial line set up, CVP/RA pressure monitoring set up, triple-lumen cardiac monitor, crash cart with defibrillator/pacemaker, nasal cannula O_2 setup, triple lumen catheter, chest tube and chest drainage system, simulated medications, 1000 mL normal saline solution, foley catheter with urometer, identification band for patient, role name tags for team members, clipboard with ICU flow sheet, lab results, 12-lead ECG results and physician's orders, telephone, code blue button.
Introduction	**Administer pre-test.** Sinus tachycardia rate of 110, BP 120/70, RR 12, SaO_2 99%, temperature 98.6°F (37°C) Pupils measure 4 mm and react briskly to light, urine 300 mL, chest tube drains 25 mL serosanguineous fluid
Body of scenario	Patient's HR progresses to 40 (second-degree heart block type 2), BP decreases to 90/40, O_2 93%, pupils: right, 4 mm, reacts briskly to light; left, 6 mm, reacts sluggishly to light, temperature 99.5°F (37.5°C); CVP 5; urine output 75 mL in last hour; chest drainage 25 mL in last hour
Conclusion	Patient's heart is successfully paced, BP improves, and improvement continues with large urine output
Debriefing	**Administer post-test.**

BP, blood pressure; RR, respiratory rate; CVP, central venous pressure.

Critical Care Simulation

Closed Head Injury Case 4.0

Scenario number: 4.0
Scenario focus: Closed Head Injury
Scenario level: Critical Care
Admission type: ICU
Patient name: Martin Neylander
Unique number: 1786807
Case number: 4.0
Date of birth: September 16, 1988
Age: 22 years
Gender: M
Attending: Ann Winters, MD
Scenario start day: Monday
Scenario start time: 0700
Admitting diagnosis: Closed head
injury
Primary diagnosis: Closed head injury
Secondary diagnosis: 1 pack per day
smoker
Recommended scenario time limit:
20–25 minutes
Recommended debriefing time limit:
20–30 minutes

Scenario purpose: Nursing management of a patient experiencing a closed head injury

Learning objectives:
The student will
1. Perform a focused assessment based on the patient's complaint or change in the patient's status.
2. Recognize normal and abnormal assessment findings.
3. Prioritize interventions based on findings and assessments.
4. Document assessment findings.
5. Perform 12-lead ECG.
6. Demonstrate nursing management of a patient experiencing a closed head injury.
7. Demonstrate ability to analyze dysrhythmias and intervene appropriately.
8. Administer medications accurately and identify indications, contraindications, and side effects associated with interventions.
9. Initiate primary ABC survey, identifying key priorities to decrease intracranial pressure.

Learning resources:
Reading assignment:
American Heart Association (2010). 2010 American heart association guidelines for cardiopulmonary resuscitation and emergency cardiovascular care. *Circulation* 122 (Suppl. 3), pp. S721, S748–S750.
Bickley, L. (2009). *Bates guide to physical assessment and history taking* (10th ed., Chapter 17). Philadelphia: Lippincott Williams & Wilkins.
Diepenbrock, N. (2012). *Quick reference to critical care* (4th ed., Chapter 1). Philadelphia: Lippincott Williams & Wilkins.
Hickey, J. (2009). *The clinical practice of neurological & neurosurgical nursing* (6th ed., Chapter 17). Philadelphia: Lippincott Williams & Wilkins.
Karch, A. (2011). *Lippincott's nursing drug guide*. Philadelphia: Lippincott Williams & Wilkins.
Morton, P., & Fontaine, D. (2010). *Critical care nursing: A holistic approach* (9th ed., Chapters 32, 33, 34, & 36.). Philadelphia: Lippincott Williams & Wilkins.
Simulation Student Workbook activities: Closed Head Injury Case 3.0 in student workbook. Student to complete pre-simulation.

RN to RN Handoff Report

Martin Neylander is a 22-year-old male patient of Dr. Winters admitted from the ER with a closed head injury as result of a cerebral contusion. He smokes a pack of cigarettes per day and drinks 3–4 beers per day. He was admitted to the ER following a motor vehicle accident. He was driving on a winding road, missed a corner, and hit a tree. He was extricated from his pickup truck with the jaws of life. He was not wearing a seatbelt. He was placed in a cervical collar and transported on a backboard to the ER. Because his Glasgow Coma Scale was 8, he was intubated with a #8 endotracheal tube by emergency medics at the scene. The initial head CT scan findings were negative. Chest x-ray demonstrated fractured ribs on the left side, with a hemothorax. A chest tube was inserted and connected to an underwater seal drainage system.

Mr. Neylander opens his eyes to painful stimuli and also withdraws all four limbs to painful stimuli. Pupils are equal and reactive to light at 4 mm. BP 120/70 mm Hg, monitor indicates sinus tachycardia 110 bpm, temperature 98.6°F (37°C), SaO_2 97% on FiO_2 0.5. Decreased breath sounds throughout left lung field. Left chest drain to −20 cm of suction, draining serosanguinous drainage. Abdomen is round and firm, hypoactive BS. Large scalp laceration was sutured in the ER. The Neylander family is in the ICU waiting room.

Mr. Neylander has no known allergies.

Blood work results and physician's orders are attached.

ER, emergency room; SaO_2, blood oxygen saturation; FiO_2, fraction of inspired oxygen; BS, bowel sounds.

Simulation Scenario

Situation/Transition	Facilitator Action	Expected Student Behavioral Outcomes	Resources
Orientation	1. Describe the setting. 2. Describe simulation experience. 3. Review simulator function (if needed).		• Simulator Directions for simulator manual

Pre-test (optional)	4. Administer pre-test.
	  a. Online quiz or
	  b. Response system (i.e., I-clickers)
			• Pre-simulation quiz attached
			• I-clicker questions

Report (see instructor script)	5. Provide report by one of the following options:
	  a. Audio
	  b. Video
	  c. Script (instructor read)
	  d. Script (student read)
		1. Student will make notes based on key points of report.	• View RN to RN Handoff report script
			• Smart phone download (audio and/or video)
			• Video

Start simulation	1. Select Scenario _____ program file. 2. Start simulation program.		• Simulator Directions for simulator manual
Phase I Introduction			
Physiologic state: HR 110 (sinus rhythm) BP (cuff) 110/70 mm Hg (arterial line) 120/70 mm Hg O_2 95% Pupils 4 mm and react briskly Temperature 98.6°F (37°C) Urine output 300 mL in past hour Chest tube to underwater seal drainage system Right radial arterial line Right internal jugular triple-lumen catheter (distal port transduced, medial port with continuous infusions, proximal port normal saline solution at 75 mL/hr) CVP 9 Ventilated on SIMV, rate 12, FiO_2 0.50, PEEP 5 cm Medications propofol 15 mcg/kg/min fentanyl 25 mcg/hr	3. Progress patient situation following Overview Recipe Card 4.0. 4. Select "Phase II Experience" from simulation software menu within 10 minutes. *Recommended time to advance:* 10 minutes	1. Student conducts systematic patient assessment, including chest drainage system and ventilator. 2. Student checks and calculates IV infusion rates for accuracy, verbalizes understanding of medications, indications, and side effects parameters to assess. 3. Student assesses hemodynamic lines, waveforms, values, and demonstrates correct method for zeroing, levelling and calibrating equipment. 4. Student demonstrates measures to decrease ICP (positioning, MAP more than 90 mm Hg, O_2 more than 92%, CVP 8–10 mm Hg, normothermia, urine output 30–200 mL/hr). 5. Student compares cuff blood pressure to intra-arterial pressure. 6. Student analyzes cardiac rhythm accurately. 7. Student uses advanced communication strategies in communicating with the ventilated patient, the patient's family, and other members of the health care team.	• Overview Recipe Card 4.0

(Continued)

Situation/Transition	Facilitator Action	Expected Student Behavioral Outcomes	Resources
		8. Student documents ventilator settings and demonstrates ability to troubleshoot alarms as they occur (low pressure). 9. Student demonstrates ability to titrate vasoactive infusions to maintain BP parameters. 10. Student notes urine output. 11. Student asks to see lab values noting CBC, electrolyte levels, BUN and creatinine results and blood glucose, urinalysis, and most recent ABG findings. 12. Student demonstrates ability to accurately interpret ABG values. 13. Student demonstrates ability to accurately interpret 12-lead ECG.	

Phase II Body of Scenario

Physiologic state: Arterial line BP 90/40 mm Hg HR 40 bpm (second-degree AV block type 2) Pupils: Right 4 mm reacts briskly, left 6 mm reacts sluggishly Temperature 99.5°F (37.5°C) SaO_2 drops to 93% CVP 5 Urine output 75 mL in past hour Chest drainage 25 mL in past hour	5. Progress patient's situation following Overview Recipe Card 4.0 6. 7. Select "Phase II Outcome" from simulation software menu within 10 minutes. *Recommended time to advance:* 5–10 minutes	1. Student recognizes MAP has decreased as a result of decreased HR 2. Student notes change in rhythm. 3. Student assesses LOC, airway, breathing. 4. Student immediately applies pacemaker pads and prepares to pace. 5. Student performs ventilator assessment. 6. Student removes blankets in response to rise in temperature. 7. Student assesses and interprets hemodynamic parameters accurately. 8. Student verbalizes potential causes for rhythm change and institutes nursing management.	• Overview Recipe Card 4.0

(Continued)

Situation/Transition	Facilitator Action	Expected Student Behavioral Outcomes	Resources
Phase III Outcome			
Physiologic state: Patient is stabilized with the use of a temporary transcutaneous pacemaker. Arterial line BP 150/70 mm Hg HR 80 bpm (ventricular paced) Pupils 5 mm react briskly to light Temperature 98.9°F (37.2°C) SaO$_2$ 98% CVP 7 Urine output 75 mL in past hour Chest drainage 25 mL in past hour	Recommended time: 5–10 minutes	1. Student conducts systematic patient assessment which includes chest drainage system and ventilator. 2. Student identifies the abnormalities in the lab results. 3. Student attempts to communicate with patient, then updates the family. 4. Student verbalizes need for collaborative intervention (temporary transvenous pacemaker).	• Simulator Directions for simulator manual
End simulation	8. End scenario. 9. Save debriefing log.		• Simulator Directions for simulator manual

HR, heart rate; SIMV, synchronized intermittent mandatory ventilation; MAP, mean arterial pressure; CBC, complete blood count; BUN, blood urea nitrogen; ABGs, arterial blood gases; PEEP, positive end-expiratory pressure; LOC, level of consciousness; ICP, intracranial pressure.

Simulation Follow-up

Situation/Transition	Instructor Action	Expected Student Behavioral Outcomes	Resources
Debriefing	1. Allow students to discuss experience. 2. Discuss student performance. 3. Watch video of simulation (optional). 4. Administer post-test. 　a. Online quiz 　b. Response system. 5. Administer post-simulation survey (optional). 6. Instruct students to complete self-evaluation/reflection (optional). 7. Provide remediation, if needed.	1. Student demonstrates ability to reflect on the scenario and discusses actions that were appropriate and interventions to modify for next time. 2. Student completes post-test	• Debriefing/Reflection Guide • Post-simulation Quiz • Simulation Student Workbook

Lab Results

Patient Identification
Martin Neylander
Unique number: 1786807

Test	Result	Normal Ranges
Chemistry Panel:		
Sodium	140	135–1425 mEq/L
Chloride	106	98–107 mEq/L
Potassium	4.3	3.5–5.1 mEq/L
Magnesium		1.3–2.1 mEq/L
BUN	12	6–20 mg/dL
		(Elderly >60 years old: 8–23 mg/dL)
Creatinine	1.1	0.4–1.3 mg/dL
Carbon dioxide, total		22–30 mEq/L
Glucose	115	62–110 mg/dL
Lactate		5–20 mg/dL
Calcium		8.6–10.3 mg/dL
HbA1C		4.0–6.7% (of total hemoglobin H)
Osmolality	300	280 to 300 mmol/kg
CBC:		
WBC	16	$4.5–11.0 \times 10^3$
RBC	4.6	Men: $4.6–6.2 \times 10^6$
		Women: $4.2–5.4 \times 10^6$
Hgb	10.0	Men: 14.0–17.4 g/dL
		Women: 12.0–16. 0 g/dL
Hct	0.36	Men: 42–52%
		Women: 37–47%
Platelets	200	$150–300 \times 10^3$

Test	Result	Marker	Normal Ranges
PT			12–14 seconds
PTT			18–28 seconds
INR			0.8–1.2
Liver Enzymes:			
ALT			7–56 U/L
ALP			38–126 U/L
Amylase			30–110 U/L
Troponin I			<0.03 ng/mL
Drug screen	Negative	Negative for opioids, benzodiazepam	
Serum lactate:			5–20 mg/dL
Arterial Blood Gases:			
Blood pH	7.33		7.34–7.44
HCO$_3$	22		22–26 mEq/L
pCO$_2$	49		35–45 mm Hg
pO$_2$	75		80–100 mm Hg
Urinalysis			
Specific gravity			1.005–1.030
Ketones		Negative	
Protein		Negative	
Leukocytes		Negative	

HbA1C, hemoglobin A1C; WBC, white blood cells; RBC, red blood cells; Hgb, hemoglobin; Hct, hematocrit; PT, prothrombin time; PTT, partial thromboplastin time; INR, international normalized ratio; ALT, alanine transaminase; ALP, alkaline phosphatase.

Hospital File

Simulation Hospital

Physician's Order Record

Patient Identification
Martin Neylander
Unquie Patient Number: 1786807

1. Use ballpoint pen.
2. Draw a line through orders not required and initial.

Admitting diagnosis: closed head injury Allergies: none known Weight: 70 kg	Code Status: Full

Monitoring:
    ✓ Record VS q15min until stable then q1h
    ✓ Continuous cardiac monitoring
    ✓ CVP q1h
    ☐ Pulmonary artery occlusive pressure q_____h
    ☐ Cardiac output/cardiac index/SVR q_____h

Activity:
    ✓ Bed rest
*elevate head of bed (HOB) 30 degrees maintain body alignment
    ☐ Position supine with HOB_____degrees
*keep HOB raised greater than 30 degrees when possible

Diet:
    ☐ Nil per os (NPO)
    ☐ Heart Smart
    ☐ 1800 kcal diabetic diet
    ✓ Enteral feedings: Insert small-bore feeding tube and commence feeding.
Type: TraumaCal rate: 10 mL/hr to start
    ✓ Consult dietitian

IV:
Total fluid to infuse 100 mL hourly
    ✓ NS at 75 mL/hr
    ☐ Lactated Ringer's at_____/hr
    ☐ D_5W at_____/hr
    ☐ Other:_____
    ✓ Hemodynamic lines to maintain patency with NS under pressure

O_2:
Titrate O_2 to maintain SaO_2 >94%
If mechanically ventilated:
ETT inserted by medics_____at 23 cm to the lip

Mode:
    ✓ _____ SIMV _____ Assist Control _____ Pressure Control _____ Pressure
    Support _____ CPAP
Rate: 12 breaths/min Tidal volume: 500 mL FiO_2: 0.50 PEEP: 5 cm
    ✓ Withhold sedation at 0600 for assessment of weaning

(Continued)

Medications:
- ☐ Aspirin, enteric coated_____mg PO daily
- ✓ Acetaminophen 650 mg PO q6h PRN pain or temperature >38.5°C
- ☐ Ceftazidime 500 mg IV q8h
- ✓ Cefazolin 1g IV q8h
- ☐ Dalteparin 5000 units SQ daily
- ☐ Furosemide_____mg IV daily
- ☐ Fentanyl__mcg q1h PRN
- ✓ Heparin 5000 units SQ q12h
- ☐ Hydromorphone 0.5–1.0 mg IV q1h PRN
- ☐ Metoprolol_____PO/ng_____
- ☐ Midazolam 2–4 mg IV q1–2h PRN
- ☐ Morphine_____IV q1–2h PRN
- ☐ Ondansetron 4 mg q__h PRN
- ✓ Phenytoin 100 mg IV q8h
- ☐ Insulin Protocol

capillary blood glucose q2h

Goal 80 to 110 mg/dL

Blood glucose = Units/hour

Less than 70 = off

70–89 = 0.2 unit/hour

90–99 = 0.5 unit/hour

100–129 = 1 unit/hour

130–179 = 1.5 unit/hour

180–239 = 2 unit/hour

240–299 = 3 unit/hour

300–359 = 4 unit/hour

>20 notify physician
- ☐ Vancomycin_____g q_____h IV

Infusions:
- ✓ Voluven 250 mL if urine output <0.5 mL/kg/hr or CVP <8 mm Hg
- ☐ Nitroglycerin 100 mg/250 mL D_5W at_____mcg/hr to max_____. Titrate for chest pain
- ✓ Dopamine 400 mg/250 mL D_5W at 3–10 mcg/kg/min titrate to maintain MAP between 70 and 105 mm Hg
- ☐ Epinephrine 2 mg/250 mL NS at_____to_____mcg/min to maintain _____greater than_____
- ☐ Dobutamine 250 mg/250 mL NS or D_5W at_____to_____to maintain _____greater than_____
- ☐ Norepinephrine 4 mg/250 mL D_5W at_____to_____maintain_____
- ☐ Vasopressin 20 U/hr_____to_____to maintain_____greater than_____
- ☐ Other:
- ✓ Propofol 100 mg/10 mL. Titrate 10 to 30 mcg/kg/min
- ✓ Fentanyl 1000 mcg/100 mL NS. Titrate 25–50 mcg/hr

Chest pain protocol:

If chest pain occurs, obtain stat ECG,
- ☐ Nitroglycerin 0.4 mg spray SL PRN for chest pain. May repeat q5min × 2 (maximum 3 doses). Then notify physician.

12-lead ECG on arrival
- ✓ Repeat ECG daily

Lab Tests:
- ☐ Albumin daily
- ☐ Bilirubin daily
- ✓ CBC daily
- ✓ Chemistry daily (electrolytes, glucose, urea, creatinine)

(Continued)

☐	Cardiac enzymes and troponin q8h × 3
✓	Cross and type 4 units
✓	ABG daily and PRN
☐	Calcium daily
☐	Magnesium daily
☐	PTT/PT daily
✓	If patient becomes febrile, obtain blood for cultures × 2

Diagnostic Tests:
- ✓ Chest x-ray (portable) daily
- ☐ Echo
- ☐ Ultrasound_____
- ✓ CT scan of head with contrast in 48 hours

Treatments:
- ✓ Daily weights
- ☐ Delirium score BID
- ☐ Change dressing as per protocol
- ☐ Physio
- ☐

Other:
- ✓ Chest tube to 20 cm of suction
- ✓ Seizure precautions

Physician's Signature:_____Date_____Time_____
Nurse's Signature:_____Date_____Time_____

Pre-and Post-test Questions

Pre-test Questions	Expected Answer /Reference
1. Describe primary and secondary injuries that occur with traumatic brain injury.	• Primary injury occurs at the time of the trauma which results in immediate damage to skull, brain structures, and main function of the particular area in the brain. • Secondary injury occurs as a result of cerebral edema, cerebral ischemia, and other cellular changes. Morton, P., & Fontaine, D. (2009). *Critical care nursing: A holistic approach* (9th ed., p. 920). Philadelphia: Lippincott Williams & Wilkins.
2. Describe acceleration–deceleration injury.	• When head hits or strikes a stationary object causing strain such as shearing or compression of cerebral tissue. Morton, P., & Fontaine, D. (2009). *Critical care nursing: A holistic approach* (9th ed., p. 921). Philadelphia: Lippincott Williams & Wilkins.
3. Explain the signs and symptoms of a patient experiencing a basal skull fracture.	• Occurs as a result of blunt force or penetration. • May occur in the anterior and middle fossae along the base of skull. • Cerebrospinal fluid draining from ear (otorrhea) may indicate a fracture in the middle fossa. • Cerebrospinal fluid draining from the nose (rhinorrhea) may indicate a fracture in the anterior fossa. • Racoon eyes and bruising behind the ears (Battle's sign) indicate a later sign of a basilar fracture. Hickey, J. (2009). *The clinical practice of neurological & neurosurgical nursing* (6th ed., p. 375). Philadelphia: Lippincott Williams & Wilkins.

Post-test Questions	Expected Answer/Reference
1. Describe the nursing management of a patient experiencing a closed head injury with potential for increased intracranial pressure.	• Oxygenation • Perfusion • Monitor neurological status • Implement measures to decrease increased intracranial pressure • Seizure prevention • Normothermia • Monitoring fluid and electrolytes • Maintaining adequate nutrition • Prevention of complications related to bed rest Morton, P., & Fontaine, D. (2009). *Critical care nursing: A holistic approach* (9th ed., p. 931). Philadelphia: Lippincott Williams & Wilkins.
2. Explain nursing actions when administering mannitol.	• Confirm physician's order • Assess current electrolytes, osmolality, ABGs, urea, and creatinine. • Monitor intake and output • Use filter when administering Hickey, J. (2009). *The clinical practice of neurological & neurosurgical nursing* (6th ed., p. 392). Philadelphia: Lippincott Williams & Wilkins.
3. Discuss nursing management of a patient experiencing diabetes insipidus.	• Thorough assessment of urine output, daily weight, changes in LOC, and vital signs • Replace urinary output with hypotonic IV solution (i.e., NS 0.45%) • Medications such as desmopressin acetate or thiazide diuretics • Monitor laboratory results (i.e., serum and urine osmolality, serum sodium, urine specific gravity) Morton, P., & Fontaine, D. (2009). *Critical care nursing: A holistic approach* (9th ed., p. 1134). Philadelphia: Lippincott Williams & Wilkins.

Competency Checklist

Closed Head Injury Case 4.0

Name: **Date:**

Competency	Examples	Met	Unmet	Comments
Performs appropriate assessment.	Comprehensive Chest drainage Focused neurological			
Demonstrates ability to correctly interpret arrhythmia and 12-lead ECG.	Sinus tachycardia Normal 12-lead ECG Second-degree heart block type 2 Paced rhythm			
Demonstrates safe management of hemodynamic monitoring.	Arterial line CVP			
Demonstrates safe management of oxygenation.	Ventilation modes Endotracheal tube			
Demonstrates safe administration of pharmacological agents.	Propofol Fentanyl			
Accurately interprets lab values.	Chemistry Hematology Drug/alcohol screen Arterial blood gases			
Demonstrates ability to quickly recognize and prioritize a patient's rapidly deteriorating condition.	Application of pacemaker			
Demonstrates principles related to safe patient care.	Alarms Lines secured Independent double checks Positioning GI prophylaxis DVT prophylaxis Seizure precautions			
Specific:	Measures to decrease intracranial pressure Identifies potential cause of large urine output Communication with team/family			

Feedback: _____
_____
_____
_____
_____

Instructor: _____

Adult Respiratory Distress Syndrome (ARDS) Case 5.0

Overview Recipe Card

Patient Name: Phillip Townsend

Scenario 5.0

Learning objectives	The student will
	1. Perform a focused assessment based on the patient's complaint or change in the patient's status.
	2. Recognize normal and abnormal assessment findings.
	3. Identify patient's worsening condition, notify physician immediately, and anticipate likely interventions for ARDS.
	4. Prioritize interventions based on findings and assessments.
	5. Document assessment findings.
	6. Demonstrate ability to analyze dysrhythmias and intervene appropriately.
	7. Administer medications accurately and identify indications, contraindications, and side effects associated with interventions.
	8. Accurately interpret arterial blood gas results and suggest potential causes and solutions.
	9. Demonstrate safe management of patient receiving neuromuscular blocking agents.
	10. Demonstrate ability to troubleshoot mechanical ventilator alarms and suggest adjustments as appropriate while managing a critically ill patient who is mechanically ventilated.
Equipment needed	Mechanical ventilator and tubing, 12-lead ECG machine, arterial line setup, peripheral IV, cardiac monitor, crash cart with defibrillator/pacemaker, rebreather face mask, manual resuscitation device and oral airway, intubation equipment, simulated medications, identification band for patient, role name tags for team members, clipboard with ICU flow sheet, lab results, 12-lead ECG results and physician's orders, telephone, code blue button, foley catheter, IV pumps, normal saline solution, and disposable bed pads.
Introduction	Administer pre-test. Mr. Townsend is an 88-year-old patient admitted from a medical floor to the ICU with an acute exacerbation of asthma. He also has a secondary diagnosis of schizophrenia.
Body of scenario	Patient is admitted with acute respiratory distress from the medical floor to the ICU. He progresses to acute respiratory failure requiring mechanical ventilation. Dopamine drip administered and titrated to keep systolic BP > 90.
Conclusion	Scenario ends with the patient stabilized and physician suggesting a family conference to discuss treatment and prognosis.
Debriefing	Administer post-test.

ARDS, adult respiratory distress syndrome; BP, blood pressure.

Critical Care Simulation

Acute Respiratory Distress Syndrome (ARDS) Case 5.0

Scenario number: 5.0
Scenario focus: ARDS
Scenario level: Critical Care
Admission type: ICU
Patient name: Phillip Townsend
Unique number: 1786808
Case number: 5.0
Date of birth: October 14, 1923
Age: 88
Gender: Male
Attending: Justine Hawkins, MD
Scenario start day: Monday
Scenario start time: 1900
Admitting diagnosis: Acute respiratory failure
Primary diagnosis: Acute respiratory failure
Secondary diagnosis: Schizophrenia
Recommended scenario time limit:
  20–25 minutes
Recommended debriefing time limit:
  20–30 minutes

Scenario purpose: Nursing management of the patient experiencing ARDS in a critical care practice setting.

Learning objectives:
The student will
  1. Perform a focused assessment based on the patient's complaint or change in the patient's status.
  2. Recognize normal and abnormal assessment findings.
  3. Identify patient's worsening condition, notify physician immediately and anticipate likely interventions for ARDS.
  4. Prioritize interventions based on findings and assessments.
  5. Document assessment findings.
  6. Demonstrate ability to analyze dysrhythmias and intervene appropriately.
  7. Administer medications accurately and identify indications, contraindications, and side effects associated with interventions.
  8. Accurately interpret arterial blood gas results.
  9. Demonstrate safe management of patient receiving neuromuscular blocking agents.
  10. Demonstrate ability to troubleshoot mechanical ventilator alarms and suggest adjustments as appropriate.

Learning resources:
Reading assignment:
  1. Morton, P., & Fontaine, D. (2009). *Critical care nursing: A holistic approach* (9th ed., Chapter 27). Philadelphia: Lippincott Williams & Wilkins.
  2. Susla, G. et al. (2006). *The handbook of critical care drug therapy* (3rd ed.). Philadelphia: Lippincott Williams and Wilkins.

Simulation Student Workbook activities: ARDS 5.0 in student workbook. Student to complete pre-simulation.

RN to RN Handoff Report
Mr. Townsend is an 88-year-old patient from a medical floor 2 days post-admission to the ICU with an acute exacerbation of asthma. He also has a secondary diagnosis of schizophrenia and tells you on admission that the "nurses on the floor were trying to kill him." He was very short of breath, very anxious, and agitated on admission to the ICU. His vital signs are as follows:

Temperature 39°C (102.2°F)

BP 140/85 mm Hg

Pulse rate 132 bpm

RR 32

O_2 saturation 89%

Face mask 0.40 FiO_2

IV normal saline solution at 100 mL/hr via right peripheral IV

Accessory muscles in use

Patient is agitated and trying to pull off face mask.

Bilateral wheezes

Extremities warm, moist, and flushed

Patient is anxious ++.

Stat ABG results show pH 7.32; pCO_2 60; HCO_3 24

The physician has just finished inserting a right radial arterial line. It has not yet been zeroed, levelled, or calibrated.

Patient has no known allergies.

His blood work results and physician's orders are attached.

RR, respiratory rate; O_2, blood oxygen saturation; FiO_2, fraction of inspired oxygen; pCO_2, partial pressure of carbon dioxide; HCO_3, bicarbonate.

Simulation Scenario Introduction

Situation/Transition	Facilitator Action	Expected Student Behavioral Outcomes	Resources
Orientation	1. Describe the setting. 2. Describe simulation experience. 3. Review simulator function (if needed).		• Simulator Directions for simulator manual

Pre-test (optional)	4. Administer pre-test.
	  a. Online quiz
	    or
	  b. Response system (i.e., I-clickers).
			• Pre-simulation quiz attached
			• I-clicker questions

Report (see instructor script)	5. Provide report by one of the following options:
	  a. Audio
	  b. Video
	  c. Script (instructor read)
	  d. Script (student read).
		1. Student makes notes based on key points of report.	• View RN to RN Handoff Report
			• Smart phone download (audio and/or video)
			• Video

Start simulation	1. Select Scenario 5.0 program file: 2. Start simulation program.		• Simulator Directions for simulator manual
Phase I Introduction			

Physiologic state:
Temperature 102.2°F (39°C)
BP 140/85 mm Hg
heart rate 132 bpm (sinus tachycardia)
RR 32
O_2 89%
Face mask .40 FiO_2 **
IV normal saline solution at 100 mL/hr
Accessory muscles in use
Patient is agitated and tries to pull off face mask
Bilateral wheezes
Extremities warm, moist, and flushed
Patient is anxious ++
Stat ABGs show
  pH 7.32
  CO_2 60
  HCO_3 24; pO_2 78
Right radial arterial line is in place
	3. Progress patient situation Overview Recipe Card 5.0
	4. Hand student second set of stat ABGs
	5. Select "Phase II Body of Scenario" from simulation software menu within 5 minutes.
	Recommended time to advance: 8 minutes
		(Temperature, tachypnea, tachycardia, decreased O_2 saturation, and signs and symptoms of respiratory distress).
		2. Student accurately analyzes arterial blood gas findings (respiratory acidosis with no compensation and mild hypoxemia).
		3. After receiving report, student performs a focused assessment based on the patient's complaint or change in the patient's status.
		4. Student recognizes abnormal assessment findings (O_2 89%, P 132, RR 32, T 39.2°C, patient anxiety, wheezing, increased work of breathing).
		5. Student states that the patient is unstable and that his condition is worsening and monitor vital signs q15min with continuous SaO_2 monitor in place.
		6. Student assists patient to be in a comfortable position, stays with the patient, gives reassurance, and explains procedures.
			• Overview Recipe Card 5.0

(Continued)

Situation/Transition	Facilitator Action	Expected Student Behavioral Outcomes	Resources
		7. Student checks blood work results and notes abnormal values (respiratory acidosis) and worsening condition. 8. Student implements prescribed interventions: • Assesses patency of IV catheter • Regulates correct IV fluid and rate • Performs ABG interpretation, and recognizes worsening respiratory acidosis). 9. Student notifies physician of patient's worsening condition and consults with respiratory therapist. 10. Student demonstrates advanced communication skills in an emergency situation with the patient, patient's family (if present), and other health care team members.	
Phase II Body of Scenario			
Physiologic state: Temperature 102.2°F (39°C) BP 88/48 Pulse rate 130 sinus tachycardia with PVCs RR 32 SaO$_2$ 89% Face mask 0.40 FiO$_2$** IV normal saline solution at 100 mL/hr Accessory muscles in use Patient is agitated and is trying to pull off mask Bilateral wheezes Extremities warm, moist, and flushed Patient is anxious ++ Patient is orally intubated with ETT and put on mechanical ventilator PSV 14 FiO$_2$ .60 PEEP 5	6. Progress patient situation following Overview Recipe Card 5.0 7. Select "Phase II Conclusion" from simulation software menu within 10 minutes. *Recommended time to advance:* 5–10 minutes	1. Student phones lab for stat ABG results (second set) or retrieves them from the chart. 2. Student assists physician with intubation and calls for stat portable chest x-ray as ordered by physician. 3. Student administers sedation and neuromuscular blocking agents as ordered observing appropriate safety measures. 4. Student troubleshoots high pressure alarms with mechanical ventilation. 5. Student provides support and explains procedures to family at bedside. 6. Student identifies complications of ARDS and signs of deterioration in patient condition. 7. Student follows procedures for VAP prevention.	• Overview Recipe Card 5.0

(Continued)

Situation/Transition	Facilitator Action	Expected Student Behavioral Outcomes	Resources
Phase III Conclusion			
Physiologic state: Patient begins to stabilize once mechanically ventilated. He is sedated and administered neuromuscular blockade. T 102.2°F (39°C) BP 88/48 P 130 sinus tachycardia with PVCs SaO_2 95% IV normal saline solution at 100 mL/hr Fine crackles in lung bases bilaterally Extremities warm and dry to touch. Patient is put on mechanical ventilator PSV 14 FiO_2 .60 PEEP 5 Family remains at bedside. Physician suggests a family conference to discuss treatment and prognosis.		1. Student demonstrates ability to provide a concise, thorough hand-off report to the oncoming shift.	• Simulator Directions for simulator manual
End simulation	8. End scenario. 9. Save debriefing log.		• Simulator Directions for simulator manual

ABGs, arterial blood gases; T, temperature; P, pulse; CO_2, carbon dioxide; pO_2, partial pressure of oxygen; PVCs, premature ventricular contractions; PSV, pressure support ventilation; PEEP, positive end-expiratory pressure; VAP, ventilator-associated pneumonia.

Simulation Follow-up

Situation/Transition	Instructor Action	Expected Student Behavioral Outcomes	Resources

Debriefing	1. Allow students to discuss experience.
	2. Discuss student performance.
	3. Watch video of simulation (optional).
	4. Administer post-test.
	  a. Online quiz.
	  b. Response system.
	5. Administer post-simulation survey (optional).
	6. Instruct students to complete self-evaluation/reflection (optional).
	7. Provide remediation, if needed.
		1. Student demonstrates ability to reflect on the scenario and discusses actions that were appropriate and interventions to modify for next time.
		2. Student completes post-test.
			• Debriefing/Reflection Guide
			• Post-simulation quiz
			• I-clicker questions
			Morton, P., & Fontaine, D. (2009). *Critical care nursing: A holistic approach* (9th ed., Chapter 27). Philadelphia: Lippincott Williams & Wilkins.
			Simulation Student Workbook ARDS follow-up questions.

Lab Results

Patient Identification
Phillip Townsend
Unique number: 1786808

Test	Result	Normal ranges
Chemistry Panel:		
Sodium	139	135–1425 mEq/L
Chloride	101	98 –107 mEq/L
Potassium	4.1	3.5–5.1 mEq/L
Magnesium		1.3–2.1 mEq/L
BUN	5.0	6–20 mg/dL
		(Elderly >60 years old: 8–23 mg/dL)
Creatinine	100	0.4–1.3 mg/dL
Carbon dioxide, total		22–30 mEq/L
Glucose	75	62–110 mg/dL
Lactate		5–20 mg/dL
Calcium		8.6–10.3 mg/dL
HbA1C		4.0–6.7% (of total hemoglobin H)
CBC:		
WBC	14.1	$4.5–11.0 \times 10^3$
RBC	4.46	Men: $4.6–6.2 \times 10^6$
		Women: $4.2–5.4 \times 10^6$
Hgb	13.8	Men: 14.0–17.4 g/dL
		Women: 12.0–16. 0 g/dL
Hct	41	Men: 42–52%
		Women: 37–47%
Platelets	200	$150–300 \times 10^3$

Test	Result	Normal ranges
PT		12–14 seconds
PTT		18–28 seconds
INR		0.8–1.2
Liver Enzymes:		
ALT	10	7–56 U/L
ALP	42	38–126 U/L
Amylase		30–110 U/L
AST	28	<35 U/L
Troponin I		<0.03 ng/mL
Serum lactate:		5–20 mg/dL
Arterial Blood Gases:		
Blood pH	7.32	7.34–7.44
HCO_3	24	22–26 mEq/L
pCO_2	60	35–45 mm Hg
pO_2	78	75–100 mm Hg

BUN, blood urea nitrogen; HbA1C, hemoglobin A1C; CBC, complete blood count; WBC, white blood cells; RBC, red blood cells; Hgb, hemoglobin; PT, prothrombin time; PTT, partial thromboplastin time; INR, international normalized ratio; ALT, alanine transaminase; ALP, alkaline phosphatase.

Simulation Hospital

Patient Identification
Phillip Townsend
Unique Patient Number: 1786808

Physician's Order Record

1. Use ballpoint pen.
2. Draw a line through orders not required and initial your changes.

Admitting Diagnosis: Acute respiratory failure Allergies: Penicillin	Code Status: Full

Monitoring:
  ✓ Record VS q15min until stable then q1h
  ✓ Continuous cardiac monitoring
  ☐ CVP q1h
  ☐ Pulmonary artery occlusive pressure q_____ h
  ☐ Cardiac output/cardiac index/SVR q_____ h	

Activity:
  ✓ Bed rest
  ✓ Position supine with HOB raised_____ degrees
*keep HOB raised more than 30 degrees when possible	

Diet:
  ☐ NPO
  ☐ Heart Smart
  ☐ 1800 kcal diabetic diet
Enteral feedings: Insert small-bore feeding tube and commence
    feeding.
Type_____ rate_____
  ✓ Consult dietitian
  ✓ Other: Full fluids	

IV:
Total fluid to infuse_____ hourly
  ✓ NS at 100 mL/h
  ☐ Lactated Ringer's at_____/h
  ☐ D_5W at_____/h
  ☐ Other:_____
  ✓ Hemodynamic lines to maintain patency with NS under pressure	

O_2: Titrate O_2 to maintain SaO_2 more than 95% If mechanically ventilated: ETT inserted by_____ at_____ cm	

Mode:
_____ SIMV_____ Assist Control_____ Pressure Support_____Pressure
  Control_____ CPAP
Rate:_____ Tidal volume_____
FiO_2_____ PEEP_____
  ☐ Withhold sedation at 0600 for assessment of weaning	

Medications:
  ☐ Aspirin, enteric coated_____ mg PO daily
  ✓ Acetaminophen 650 mg PO q6h PRN for pain or temperature
    over 38.5°C
  ☐ Ceftazidime 500 mg IV q8h
  ☐ Cefazolin 1g IV q8h	

(Continued)

☐ Dalteparin 5000 units SQ daily
☐ Furosemide_____ mg IV daily
☐ Fentanyl_____ mcg q1h PRN
☐ Heparin 5000 units SQ q12h
☐ Hydromorphone 0.5–1.0 mg IV q1h PRN
☐ Metoprolol_____ PO/ng_____
☐ Midazolam 2–4 mg IV q1–2h PRN
✓ Morphine 2–4mg IV q1–2h PRN
☐ Ondansetron 4 mg q_____h PRN
☐ Insulin Protocol
capillary blood glucose q2h
Goal 80 to 110 mg/dL
Blood glucose = Units/hour
Less than 70 = off
70–89 = 0.2 unit/hour
90–99 = 0.5 unit/hour
100–129 = 1 unit/hour
130–179 = 1.5 unit/hour
180–239 = 2 unit/hour
240–299 = 3 unit/hour
300–359 = 4 unit/hour
>20 notify physician
☐ Vancomycin_____ g q_____ h IV
✓ Other: Albuterol 1.25–5 mg every 1–4 hours as needed
✓ Prednisone IV 40 mg BID
✓ Atrovent 0.5 mg PRN

Infusions:
☐ Voluven _____ mL if urine output less than 0.5 mL/kg/h or CVP less than _____
☐ Nitroglycerin 100 mg/250 mL D_5W at_____ mcg/h to max _____ . Titrate for chest pain.
☐ Dopamine 200 mg/250 mL D_5W at_____ to_____ titrate to maintain _____ greater than _____
☐ Epinephrine 2 mg/250 mL NS at_____ to_____ mcg/min to maintain _____ greater than _____
☐ Dobutamine 250 mg/250 mL NS or D_5W at_____ to_____ to maintain _____ greater than _____
☐ Norepinephrine 4 mg/250 mL D_5W at_____ to_____ maintain _____
☐ Vasopressin 20 U/h _____ to _____ to maintain _____ greater than _____
☐ Other:

Chest pain protocol:
If chest pain occurs, obtain stat ECG.
☐ Nitroglycerin 0.4 mg spray SL PRN for chest pain. May repeat q5min × 2 (maximum 3 doses). Then notify physician

12-lead ECG on arrival
✓ Repeat ECG daily

Lab tests:
☐ Albumin daily
☐ Bilirubin daily
✓ CBC daily
✓ Chemistry daily (electrolytes, glucose, urea, creatinine)
☐ Cardiac enzymes and troponin q8h × 3
☐ Cross and type _____ units
✓ ABG daily and PRN
☐ Calcium daily

(Continued)

☐ Magnesium daily
☐ PTT/PT daily
✓ If patient becomes febrile, obtain blood for culture × 2
✓ Sputum for C & S
Diagnostic tests:
✓ Chest x-ray (portable) daily
☐ Echo
☐ Ultrasound _____
☐ CT scan _____
Treatments:
☐ Daily weights
✓ Delirium score BID
☐ Change dressing as per protocol
☐ Physio

Other:

Physician's Signature:_____ Date_____ Time_____
Nurse's Signature:_____ Date_____ Time_____

Pre- and Post-Test Questions

Pre-test Questions	Expected Answer/Reference
1. Discuss some of the potential causes of ARDS.	1. **Direct injury** (e.g., chest trauma–pulmonary contusion, near drowning, hypervolemia–pulmonary edema, inhalation of toxic gases and vapors–smoke chemicals, oxygen toxicity, pneumonia, aspiration pneumonitis, radiation pneumonitis, pulmonary embolism—especially amniotic or fat, radiation, and drugs (e.g., bleomycin). 2. **Indirect injury:** Sepsis (most likely cause), shock, multisystem trauma, burns, cardiopulmonary bypass, disseminated intravascular coagulation, toxemia of pregnancy, acute pancreatitis, diabetic coma, central nervous system injury, drug over dosage, blood transfusion, and abdominal trauma. Dennison, R. (2007). *Pass CCRN!*, Mosby, St. Louis. (p. 313). Morton, P., & Fontaine, D. (2009). *Critical care nursing: A holistic approach* (9th ed., p. 672). Philadelphia: Lippincott Williams & Wilkins.
2. In ARDS, a refractory hypoxemia develops as one of the hallmark characteristics. What does this mean?	Refractory hypoxemia refers to the condition in which hypoxemia worsens (PaO_2 does not improve) despite intervening with additional supplemental oxygen. Morton, P., & Fontaine, D. (2009). *Critical care nursing: A holistic approach* (9th ed., p. 678). Philadelphia: Lippincott Williams & Wilkins.
3. What is the main goal of treatment in ARDS?	The main goal of treatment is to improve oxygenation and ventilation Morton, P., & Fontaine, D. (2009). *Critical care nursing: A holistic approach* (9th ed., p. 680). Philadelphia: Lippincott Williams & Wilkins.

Post-test Questions	Expected Answer/Reference
1. Describe types of pharmacological interventions that may be used as supportive treatment in ARDS.	Pharmacological treatment in ARDS is supportive. Some medications that may be used over the course are • Antibiotics (in the presence of a known microorganism). • Bronchodilators and mucolytics. • Corticosteroids. Morton, P., & Fontaine, D. (2009). *Critical care nursing: A holistic approach* (9th ed., p. 682). Philadelphia: Lippincott Williams & Wilkins.
2. Why is early nutritional support essential in patients experiencing ARDS?	Early enteral feedings speed recovery in ARDS patients since protein loss is prevented and mortality rates are decreased. Morton, P., & Fontaine, D. (2009). *Critical care nursing: A holistic approach* (9th ed., p. 683). Philadelphia: Lippincott Williams & Wilkins.
3. What types of interventions can help prevent complications in ARDS?	Avoiding mechanical ventilation with high levels of PEEP, high tidal volumes, and volume controlled modes will assist in preventing complications of ARDS, such as volutrauma and barotraumas, which can lead to other complications (e.g., pneumothorax). Other complications can include DVT due to immobility, VAP and aspiration from enteral feedings, therefore VAP precautions need to be followed, head of bed elevated with administration of enteral feeds and passive and active range of motion exercises to prevent DVT. Morton, P., & Fontaine, D. (2009). *Critical care nursing: A holistic approach* (9th ed., p. 683). Philadelphia: Lippincott Williams & Wilkins.

DVT, deep vein thrombosis.

Competency Checklist

ARDS Case 5.0

Name: **Date:**

Competency	Examples	Met	Unmet	Comments
Performs appropriate assessment.	Emergency Comprehensive			
12- and 15-lead ECG proficiency.	Performs 12-lead ECG 12-lead ECG interpretation Performs 15-lead ECG			
Demonstrates ability to correctly interpret arrhythmia	• Sinus tachycardia with PVCs			
Demonstrates safe management of hemodynamic monitoring.	Pulmonary artery catheter CVP/PAOP/PCWP Cardiac output Arterial catheter			
Demonstrates safe management of oxygenation.	Ventilation modes Arterial Blood Gas interpretation Troubleshoots ventilator alarms			
Demonstrates safe administration of pharmacological agents. Accurately interprets lab values.	Dopamine infusion Sedation administration Chemistry Hematology Arterial blood gases			
Demonstrates ability to quickly recognize and prioritize a patient's rapidly deteriorating condition.	Hypotension Decreased level of consciousness Assessment of respiratory distress			
Demonstrates principles related to safe patient care.	Alarms on Accurate hand-off report			
Specific:	Communication with patient and health care team Lines secured Independent double checks Positioning Communication with family Able to suggest anticipated ventilator changes based on ABGs and changing patient's condition Suctions ETT as appropriate Follows best practice guidelines for VAP prevention			

Feedback: _____

_____

_____

_____

_____

Instructor: _____

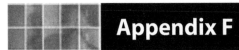

Renal Failure Case 6.0

Overview Recipe Card

Patient Name: Anthony Liu

Scenario 6.0

Learning objectives	**The student will** 1. Perform a focused assessment based on the patient's complaint or change in the patient's status. 2. Recognize normal and abnormal assessment findings. 3. Prioritize interventions based on findings and assessments. 4. Document assessment findings. 5. Demonstrate appropriate management of hemodynamic lines. 6. Demonstrate ability to systematically interpret dysrhythmias related to patient's condition. 7. Demonstrate ability to analyze lab data and integrate the data with patient assessment. 8. Administer medications accurately and identify indications, contraindications, and side effects associated with interventions. 9. Call for team assistance as appropriate. 10. Initiate primary ABC measures and safely initiate appropriate interventions related to a hypotensive crisis.
Equipment needed	12-lead ECG machine, pressure monitoring set with 2 flush systems for arterial pressure and central venous pressure, triple-lumen catheter, cardiac monitor, crash cart with cardioversion capabilities, manual resuscitation device, oral airway, disposable gloves, simulated medications, 250 mL normal Saline solution, IV pole, Mefix dressing for sternum and left leg, Foley catheter with urometer, identification band for patient, role name tags for team, clip board with ICU flow sheet, lab results, 12-lead ECG results and physician's orders, telephone, and code blue button.
Introduction	**Administer pre-test.**
Body of scenario	Two days post-quadruple bypass surgery, the patient experiences renal failure (hyperkalemia, diminishing urinary output, peripheral edema). The patient's condition changes when he develops an unstable ventricular tachycardia with a pulse rate requiring the nurse, to prepare for immediate cardioversion.
Conclusion	Nurse updates patient's family regarding the cardioversion and the potential for renal dialysis.
Debriefing	**Administer post-test.**

Critical Care Simulation

Renal Failure Case 6.0

Scenario number: 6.0
Scenario focus: Renal failure
Scenario level: Critical care
Admission type: ICU
Patient name: Anthony Liu
Unique number: 1786809
Case number: 6.0
Date of birth: June 2, 1946
Age: 65
Gender: M
Attending: Bernard Cohen, MD
Scenario start day: Monday
Scenario start time: 0700
Admitting diagnosis:
Coronary artery disease
Primary diagnosis: Aortic coronary bypass grafting × 4
Secondary diagnosis:
NIDDM, renal insufficiency, hypertension
Recommended scenario time limit: 20–25 minutes
Recommended debriefing time limit: 20–30 minutes

Scenario purpose: Nursing management of the post-bypass patient experiencing renal failure and subsequent hypotensive episode in a critical care practice setting.

Learning objectives:
The student will
1. Perform a focused assessment based on the patient's complaint or change in the patient's status.
2. Recognize normal and abnormal assessment findings.
3. Prioritize interventions based on findings and assessments.
4. Document assessment findings.
5. Demonstrate accurate management of hemodynamic lines.
6. Demonstrate ability to systematically interpret dysrhythmias as related to patient's condition.
7. Demonstrate ability to analyze lab data and integrate the data with patient assessment.
8. Administer medications accurately and identify indications, contraindications, and side effects associated with interventions.
9. Call for assistance of team members as appropriate.
10. Initiate primary ABC measures and safely initiate appropriate interventions related to a hypotensive crisis.
11. Demonstrate ability to provide a concise, thorough, hand-off report to the oncoming shift.

Learning resources:
Reading assignment:
American Heart Association (2010). 2010 American heart association guidelines for cardiopulmonary resuscitation and emergency cardiovascular care. *Circulation* 122 (Suppl. 3):S685–S719.
Bickley, L. (2009). *Bates guide to physical assessment and history taking* (10th ed., Chapter 17). Philadelphia: Lippincott Williams & Wilkins.
Diepenbrock, N. (2012). *Quick reference to critical care* (4th ed., Chapter 1). Philadelphia: Lippincott Williams & Wilkins.
Hickey, J. (2009). *The clinical practice of neurological & neurosurgical nursing* (6th ed., Chapter 17). Philadelphia: Lippincott Williams & Wilkins.
Karch, A. (2011). *Lippincott's nursing drug guide.* Philadelphia: Lippincott Williams & Wilkins.
Morton, P., & Fontaine, D. (2010). *Critical care nursing: A holistic approach* (9th ed., Chapters 32, 33, 34, & 36). Philadelphia: Lippincott Williams & Wilkins.
Simulation Student Workbook activities: Renal failure 6.0 in student workbook. Student to complete pre-simulation.

RN to RN Handoff Report

Anthony Liu is a 65-year-old male patient of Dr. Cohen. He was admitted from the cardiac OR after undergoing coronary artery bypass grafting of four vessels 2 days ago. He has a history of hypertension, non–insulin-dependent diabetes controlled on glyburide, and elevated creatinine levels. Mr. Liu recently quit smoking, after smoking a packet of cigarettes per day for over 20 years. Medications at home include metoprolol 50 mg daily, amlodipine 5 mg daily, atorvastatin 20 mg daily, glyburide 5 mg daily with breakfast, and nitroglycerin spray PRN. Currently Mr. Liu is lethargic but easily rouses to name; pain is managed with two tablets of Percocet q4h; BP has ranged from 95/60 mm Hg to 110/60 mm Hg, sinus rhythm with frequent PVCs, all pulses are weak, but palpable, skin is dry, extremities cool to touch, large amount of pitting edema. CVP ranges from 10 to 15 mm Hg. Mr. Liu is receiving FiO$_2$ 0.40 per face mask with coarse crackles scattered throughout the lungs; he has a weak, nonproductive cough; sternal dressings and left leg dressings (graft site) are dry and intact, urine output has been low postoperatively, ranging from 10 to 25 mL/h of dark amber urine. His fluid balance is 3000 mL positive since the OR 2 days ago. To improve Mr. Liu's urine output, he has received several doses of IV furosemide boluses of 80 mg and is now receiving a furosemide infusion at 10 mg/h. He has also received two doses metolazone10 mg for diminishing urine output. Abdomen is soft and bowel sounds are occasional; therefore, he receives only sips of fluids. He has a triple-lumen catheter via right internal jugular vein with distal port transduced, medial port and proximal port have normal saline solution infusing to keep vein open, regular insulin 100 units in 100 mL of NS is infusing at 2 units per hour via proximal port right radial arterial line transduced.

He has environmental allergies.

Blood work results and physician's orders are attached.

NIDDM, non–insulin-dependent diabetes mellitus; OR, operating room; PVC, premature ventricular contraction; CVP, central venous pressure

Simulation Scenario

Situation/Transition	Facilitator Action	Expected Student Behavioral Outcomes	Resources
Orientation	1. Describe the setting 2. Describe simulation experience 3. Review simulator function (if needed)		• Simulator Directions for simulator manual

Pre-test (optional)	4. Administer pre-test
	  a. Online quiz
	    or
	  b. Response system (i.e., I-clickers)
			• Pre-simulation quiz attached
			• I-clicker questions

Report (see instructor script)	5. Provide report by one of the following options:
	  a. Audio
	  b. Video
	  c. Script (instructor read)
	  d. Script (student read).
		1. Student will make notes based on key points of report.	• View RN handoff report script
			• Smart phone download (audio and/or video)
			• Video

Start simulation	1. Select scenario___ program file 2. Start simulation program. Set up vital signs and beginning of patient parameters.		• Simulator Directions for simulator manual
Phase I Introduction			
Physiologic state: HR 98 (sinus rhythm with peaked T wave and frequent PVCs) SaO_2 94% on FiO_2 0.40 per facemask Right radial arterial line with normal arterial waveform (BP) 95/60 mm Hg; cuff BP 95/60 mm Hg Temperature 96.8°F (36°C) CVP transduced via distal port of right triple-lumen catheter with normal waveform CVP 15 mm Hg Normal saline solution TKVO via medial and distal ports; right triple-lumen catheter Furosemide 100 mg/100 mL normal saline solution at 10 mL/h via medial port (light protected) Regular insulin 100 units in 100 mL of NS is infusing at 2 units per hour via proximal port Urine output 10 mL dark amber urine	3. Progress patient situation following Overview Recipe Card 6.0 *Recommended time to advance scenario:* 10 minutes	1. Student conducts systematic patient assessment noting abnormal findings. 2. Student checks orders and lab values, and calculates IV infusion rates for accuracy, verbalizes understanding of medications, indications and side effects parameters to assess. 3. Student demonstrates ability to assess and manage all hemodynamic lines, waveforms, and values and knows the correct method for zeroing, leveling and calibrating equipment. 4. Student compares cuff blood pressure to intra-arterial pressure. 5. Student analyzes cardiac rhythm accurately and notes peaked T wave. 6. Student uses advanced communication strategies for communicating with the anxious patient, the patient's family, and other members of the health care team. 7. Student documents accurately on ICU flow sheet. 8. Student demonstrates ability to accurately interpret blood work and recognizes abnormal values.	• Overview Recipe Card 6.0

Situation/Transition	Facilitator Action	Expected Student Behavioral Outcomes	Resources
Phase II Body of Scenario			
Physiologic state: Blood pressure drops 72/42 mm Hg HR 180 (supraventricular tachycardia) CVP 15 mm Hg Chest: coarse crackles SaO$_2$ 81% on FiO$_2$ 0.40 per facemask Patient responds to noxious/painful stimuli only After cardioversion, the rhythm changes to sinus rhythm 90 bpm (with peaked T waves) BP 90/60 mm Hg RR 12 bpm	4. Progress patient situation following Overview Recipe Card 6.0 • Select "Phase II Outcome" from simulation software menu within 10 minutes. *Recommended time to advance scenario:* 8 minutes Provide student with second stat lab results	1. Student demonstrates ability to recognize life-threatening dysrhythmias and calls physician stat. 2. Student notes decreased blood pressure and patient's instability and immediately calls for help. Student requests physician stat, draws blood for ABG and electrolyte analysis, and prepares for cardioversion. 3. Student changes FiO$_2$ apparatus to bag–valve–mask and monitors respirations. 4. Physician arrives to perform cardioversion for patient at 100 joules. 5. Student identifies current rhythm correctly as sinus rhythm with peaked T waves and continues to assess BP and RR. 6. Student interprets second set of lab results accurately and suggests the antidote for hyperkalemia as the treatment of choice (e.g., calcium gluconate 1 g IV, regular insulin 10 units IV and D$_{50}$W 1 ampule). 7. In collaboration with team, student suggests nephrology consult for potential CRRT	• Overview Recipe Card 6.0
Phase III Conclusion of Scenario			
Physiologic state: Arterial line BP 95/60 mm Hg Sinus rhythm with peaked T waves 95 bpm CVP 15 mm Hg Chest: fewer crackles throughout SaO$_2$ 94% *End simulation*	*Recommended time to advance scenario:* 5 minutes	1. Student uses advanced communication skills with family regarding cardiac dysrhythmias requiring cardioversion, as well as potential for patient to require dialysis. 2. Student completes reassessment and documentation.	Prepare to go to debriefing session.

HR, heart rate; PVC, premature ventricular contraction; SaO$_2$, blood oxygen saturation; FiO$_2$, fraction of inspired oxygen; BP, blood pressure; CVP, central venous pressure; TKVO, to keep vein open; ABG, arterial blood gas; RR, respiratory rate; CRRT, continuous renal replacement therapy.

Simulation Follow-up

Situation/Transition	Instructor Action	Expected Student Behavioral Outcomes	Resources
Debriefing	1. Allow students to discuss experience 2. Discuss student performance 3. Watch video of simulation (optional) 4. Administer post-test (attached) a. Online quiz b. Response system 5. Administer post-simulation survey (optional) 6. Instruct students to complete self-evaluation/reflection (optional) 7. Provide remediation, if needed.	1. Student demonstrates ability to reflect on the scenario and discusses actions that were appropriate and interventions to modify for next time. 2. Student completes post-test.	• I-clicker questions • Post-test Simulation Student Workbook follow-up assignment.

Lab Results (Scene 1)

Patient Identification
Anthony Liu
Unique number: 1786809

Test	Result	Normal Ranges
Chemistry panel:		
Sodium	133	135–1425 mEq/L
Chloride	110	98–107 mEq/L
Potassium	6.4	3.5–5.1 mEq/L
Magnesium	2.2	1.3–2.1 mEq/L
BUN	21	6–20 mg/dL
		(Elderly >60 years old: 8–23 mg/dL)
Creatinine	5	0.4–1.3 mg/dL
Carbon dioxide, total	18	22–30 mEq/L
Glucose	135	62–110 mg/dL
Lactate		5–20 mg/dL
Calcium	7	8.6–10.3 mg/dL
Ionized calcium		4.8–5.2 mg/dL
Phosphorus	1.45	2.4–5.1 mg/dL
HbA1C	7	4.0–6.7% (of total hemoglobin H)
CBC:		
WBC	13	$4.5–11.0 \times 10^3$
RBC	4.2	Men: $4.6–6.2 \times 10^6$
		Women: $4.2–5.4 \times 10$
Hgb	90	Men: 14.0–17.4 g/dL
		Women: 12.0–16.0 g/dL
Hct	41	Men: 42–52%
		Women: 37–47%
Platelets	100	$150–300 \times 10^3$

BUN, blood urea nitrogen; CBC, complete blood count; WBC, white blood cells; RBC, red blood cells; Hgb, hemoglobin; hct, hematocrit.

Test	Result	Normal Ranges
PT		12–14 seconds
PTT	38	18–28 seconds
INR	1.2	0.8–1.2
Liver enzymes:		
ALT	22	7–56 U/L
ALP		38–126 U/L
Amylase		30–110 U/L
Troponin I	0.03	<0.03 ng/ml
Serum lactate:		5–20 mg/dL
Arterial Blood Gases:		
Blood pH	7.33	7.34–7.44
HCO_3	18	22–26 mEq/L
pCO_2	33	35–45 mm Hg
pO_2	70	75–100 mm Hg

PT, prothrombin time; PTT, partial thromboplastin time; INR, international normalized ratio; ALT, alanine transaminase; ALP, Alkaline phosphatase.

Stat Lab Results

Preliminary Results Scene 3

Date/Time:_____Patient Name:_____Anthony Liu_____

Hematology	Chemistry
Hgb_____Hct:_____ WBC:_____Platelets:_____ Other:	Na:_____131 K: 6.2 Cl: 110 HCO₃: 17 Urea: 21 Creatinine: 390 Glucose:_____ CPK:_____Troponin:_____ AST:_____ALT:_____ Other: ABGs: pH 7.33, pCO₂ 39, pO₂ 75, HCO₃ 16
Coagulation studies PT:_____PTT:_____ INR:_____ Bleeding time:_____ D-dimers:_____ Fibrin split products:_____ Other:	**Urinalysis** pH:_____ Glucose:_____ Ketones:_____ Specific gravity:_____ Blood:_____ Protein:_____ Leukocyte:_____

Hgb, hemoglobin; WBC, white blood cells; CPK, creatine phosphokinase; ALT, alanine transaminase; ALP, Alkaline phosphatase; ABGs, arterial blood gases.

Patient Identification
Anthony G. Lui
Unique Patient Number: 1786807
Hospital File

Simulation Hospital

Physician's Order Record

1. Use ballpoint pen.
2. Draw a line through orders not required and initial.

Admitting Diagnosis: CABG × 4 Allergies: Environmental	Code Status: Full
Monitoring: ✓ Record VS Q15 minutes until stable then q1h ✓ Continuous cardiac monitoring ☐ CVP q1h ☐ Pulmonary artery occlusive pressure q_____ h ☐ Cardiac output/cardiac index/SVR q_____ h	
Activity: ✓ Bedrest ✓ Position supine with HOB raised_____ degrees *keep HOB raised more than 30 degrees when possible ✓ Ambulate with physiotherapist	

(Continued)

Diet:
- ☐ NPO
- ✓ Heart Smart
- ☐ 1800 kcal diabetic diet
- ☐ Enteral feedings: Insert small bore feeding tube and commence feedings.

Type _____ Rate _____
- ✓ Consult dietician re: nephrology diet

IV:

Total fluid to infuse 50 mL hourly
- ✓ NS at 50/hr
- ☐ Lactated Ringer's at _____ /hr
- ☐ D_5W at _____ /hr
- ☐ Other:_____
- ✓ Hemodynamic lines to maintain patency with NS under pressure

O_2:
- ✓ Titrate O_2 to maintain SaO_2 greater than 94%

If mechanically ventilated:

ETT inserted by_____ at _____ cm

Mode:

_____ SIMV_____ Assist Control _____ Pressure Support _____Pressure

Control _____ CPAP

Rate:_____ Tidal volume _____

FiO_2_____ PEEP_____
- ☐ Withhold sedation at 0600 for assessment of weaning

Medications:
- ✓ Aspirin, enteric coated 325 mg PO daily
- ✓ Acetaminophen 650 mg PO q6h PRN for pain or temp more than 38.5°C celsius
- ☐ Ceftazidime 500 mg IV q8h
- ✓ Cefazolin 1g IV q8h
- ☐ Dalteparin 5000 units SQ daily
- ✓ Furosemide <u>reassess</u> IV daily
- ✓ Fentanyl 25 mcg q1h PRN
- ✓ Heparin 5000 units SQ q12h
- ☐ Hydromorphone 0.5–1.0 mg IV q1h PRN
- ✓ Metoprolol 25 PO/ng daily (hold if SPB less than 100 mm Hg)
- ☐ Midazolam 2–4 mg IV q1–2h PRN
- ✓ Morphine 2–4mg IV q1–2h PRN
- ✓ Ondansetron 4 mg q_____h PRN
- ✓ Percocet 1 or 2 tabs PO q4h PRN for pain

  Insulin Protocol

capillary blood glucose q2h

Goal 80 to 110 mg/dL

Blood glucose = Units/hour

Less than 70 = off

70–89 = 0.2 unit/hour

90–99 = 0.5 unit/hour

100–129 = 1 unit/hour

130–179 = 1.5 unit/hour

180–239 = 2 unit/hour

240–299 = 3 unit/hour

300–359 = 4 unit/hour

Greater than 20 notify physician
- ☐ Vancomycin_____ g q_____ h IV

(Continued)

Infusions:

☐ Voluven_____mL if urine output less than 0.5 mL/kg/h or CVP less than_____

☐ Nitroglycerin 100 mg/250 mL D_5W at _____ mcg/h to max_____ . Titrate for chest pain

☐ Dopamine 200 mg/250 mL D_5W at _____ to_____ titrate to maintain_____ greater than_____

☐ Epinephrine 2 mg/250 mL NS at _____ to_____ mcg/min to maintain_____ greater than_____

☐ Dobutamine 250 mg/250 mL NS or D_5W at _____ to_____ to maintain_____ greater than_____

☐ Norepinephrine 4 mg/250 mL D_5W at _____ to_____ maintain_____

☐ Vasopressin 20 U/h_____ to _____ to maintain_____ greater than_____

☐ Other:

✓ Lasix 100 mg/100 mL NS at 10 mL/hr

Chest pain protocol:

If chest pain occurs, obtain stat ECG.

☐ Nitroglycerin 0.4 mg spray SL PRN for chest pain. May repeat q5 min × 2 (maximum 3 doses). Then notify physician

---

12-lead ECG on arrival

☐ Repeat ECG q8h × 2

✓ ECG daily

Lab Tests:

☐ Albumin daily

☐ Bilirubin daily

✓ CBC daily

✓ Chemistry BID (electrolytes, glucose, urea, creatinine)

☐ Cardiac enzymes and troponin q8h × 3

☐ Cross and type_____ units

✓ ABG daily and PRN

✓ Calcium daily

✓ Magnesium daily

✓ PTT/PT daily

✓ If patient becomes febrile, obtain blood for culture × 2

Diagnostic Tests:

✓ Chest x-ray (portable) daily

☐ Echo

☐ Ultrasound_____

☐ CT scan_____

Treatments:

✓ Daily weights

✓ Delirium score BID

✓ Change dressing as per protocol

✓ Physio

Other:

Nephrology to see

Physician's Signature:_____Date_____Time_____

Nurse's Signature:_____Date_____Time_____

Pre- and Post-test Questions

Pre-test Questions	Expected Answer/Reference
1. Discuss one classification or presentation of renal failure (prerenal, intrarenal, and postrenal) and identify a precipitating condition or cause.	**Prerenal causes of renal failure (ARF):** Decreased circulating volume (dehydration, hemorrhage, hypovolemic shock, third-spacing fluids); cardiac failure (congestive heart failure, myocardial infarction, cardiogenic shock, valvular heart disease); medications (ACE inhibitors, NSAIDs), decreased renal perfusion (sepsis, cirrhosis, neurogenic shock) **Intrarenal causes of ARF:** Acute glomerulonephritis (immune disorder, vasculitis), vascular disease (scleroderma, atheroembolic event), acute interstitial disease, acute pyelonephritis, tubular obstruction, multiple myeloma, ATN from ischemia (hypotension, volume depletion or cardiac surgery), or ATN from nephrotoxic agents, such as antimicrobials or contrast media, heme pigments or chemicals, such as pesticides or organic solvents. **Postrenal causes of ARF:** Any obstruction in urine flow may cause an obstruction. Renal calculi, urethral or ureteral strictures, BPH are causes of postrenal ARF. Morton, P., & Fontaine, D. (2009). *Critical care nursing: A holistic approach* (9th ed., p. 759). Philadelphia: Lippincott Williams & Wilkins.
2. Identify one of the four phases of ATN and identify a nursing priority for each.	The **onset phase** begins with the initial onset lasting hours to days, identified by the increase in serum creatinine level. The next phase, **oliguric or nonoliguric phase,** lasts approximately 1 week. If the precipitating event is due to ischemia, the patient becomes oliguric which typically lasts 7–14 days. Patients presenting with oliguric ATN may develop fluid overload, electrolyte abnormality, and metabolic acidosis. Nonoliguric phase which may last 5–7 days, is associated with a toxic injury (e.g., from contrast media). As the kidney is unable to concentrate the urine, large volumes of urine are excreted. The complications associated with nonoliguric ATN are electrolyte abnormalities, specifically hyperkalemia. The **diuretic phase** lasts 1–2 weeks, as the kidneys slowly regain function. The kidneys can excrete up to 10 liters daily; however, function may still be impaired. Monitoring of electrolyte abnormalities, such as hyponatremia and hypokalemia, is required. The **recovery phase** may take several months to a year. The patient may experience full or near-full recovery of renal function. Education of the patient to preserve renal function (diet, medications, monitoring kidney function, monitoring blood pressure, and fluid overload). Morton, P., & Fontaine, D. (2009). *Critical care nursing: A holistic approach* (9th ed., pp. 764–765). Philadelphia: Lippincott Williams & Wilkins.
3. Discuss the role of a dopamine infusion in ARF.	Dopamine is a vasoactive inotrope at higher doses and can stimulate dopaminergic receptors at lower levels to induce renal blood flow. There is lack of evidence to support this infusion practice in preventing ARF or improving patient outcomes. Morton, P., & Fontaine, D. (2009). *Critical care nursing: A holistic approach* (9th ed., p. 748, 775). Philadelphia: Lippincott Williams & Wilkins.

ARF, acute renal failure; ACE, angiotensin-converting enzyme; NSAIDs, nonsteroidal anti-inflammatory drugs; ATN, acute tubular necrosis; BPH, benign prostatic hypertrophy.

Post-test Questions	Expected Answer/Reference
1. What are the important lab and diagnostic tests to be monitored when a patient experiences ARF?	The urinalysis would provide information about the sodium concentration, urine specific gravity, and sediment in the urine. Depending on the results obtained, helps to identify whether the renal failure was prerenal or intrarenal. Blood urea nitrogen and creatinine values are closely monitored not only for an increase, but also for the proportionate relationship. Monitor electrolytes for hyperkalemia, as well as arterial blood gas values for metabolic acidosis. Diagnostic tests useful in monitoring renal status are renal ultrasound, CT, and MRI. Morton, P., & Fontaine, D. (2009). *Critical care nursing: A holistic approach* (9th ed., pp. 766–767). Philadelphia: Lippincott Williams & Wilkins.
2. Describe key priorities in the nursing management of ARF according to classification (e.g., prerenal, intrarenal, and postrenal).	Management of prerenal renal failure begins with thorough assessment of the patient, looking for signs of hypovolemia. Restoring the intravascular volume, with NS IV boluses or blood replacement as required. Management of intrarenal renal failure causing ATN is treated initially with diuretics and fluids to flush tubules of cellular casts. Discontinue any nephrotoxic drugs; adjust dosage according to laboratory values. Postrenal management involves removing obstruction. Morton, P., & Fontaine, D. (2009). *Critical care nursing: A holistic approach* (9th ed., pp. 771–784). Philadelphia: Lippincott Williams & Wilkins.
3. Discuss the indications and contraindications for CRRT.	CRRT is indicated for patients who have the potential to develop acute hemodynamic compromise and who are unable to tolerate hemodialysis. These patients require drug or toxin removal, excess fluid removal as well as electrolyte and acid–base corrections. Contraindications for CRRT include a patient's coagulopathies or severe vascular disease that make access difficult. Morton, P., & Fontaine, D. (2009). *Critical care nursing: A holistic approach* (9th ed., p. 737). Philadelphia: Lippincott Williams & Wilkins. Diepenbrock, N. (2012). *Quick reference to critical care* (4th ed., pp. 51–52, 251). Philadelphia: Lippincott, Williams & Wilkins.

ARF, acute renal failure; ATN, acute tubular necrosis; CRRT, continuous renal replacement therapy.

Competency Checklist

Renal Failure Case 6.0

Name: **Date:**

Competency	Examples	Met	Unmet	Comments
Performs appropriate assessment	Comprehensive Focused respiratory			
Demonstrates ability to correctly interpret arrhythmia and 12-lead ECG	Sinus rhythm with premature ventricular contractions and peaked T waves SVT			
Demonstrates safe management of hemodynamic monitoring	Arterial line CVP			
Demonstrates safe management of oxygenation	Airway management during cardioversion			
Demonstrates safe administration of pharmacological agents	Lasix infusion Midazolam			
Accurately interprets lab values	Chemistry/glucose Hematology Arterial blood gases Urea/creatinine			
Demonstrates ability to quickly recognize and prioritize a patient's rapidly deteriorating condition	Synchronized cardioversion Draws labs from arterial line			
Demonstrates principles related to safe patient care	Alarms Lines secured Independent double checks Positioning Handover report			
Specific	Diabetes management Treatment for hyperkalemia Handover report Communication with patient/family/team Anticipates CRRT			

Feedback:_____
_____
_____
_____
_____
_____

Instructor:_____

Liver Failure Case 7.0

Overview Recipe Card

Patient Name: Daniel Arthur Adams

Scenario 7.0

Learning objectives	The student will
	1. Perform a focused assessment based on the patient's complaint or change in the patient's status.
	2. Recognize normal and abnormal assessment findings.
	3. Recognize abnormal lab values related to liver failure.
	4. Prioritize interventions based on findings and assessments.
	5. Document assessment findings.
	6. Recognize and manage complications associated with liver failure.
	7. Discuss rationale for medications and diagnostics ordered in the patient experiencing acute liver failure.
	8. Recognize signs of respiratory distress and impending respiratory failure and intervene appropriately.
	9. Demonstrate ability to analyze arrhythmias and intervenes appropriately.
Equipment needed	12-lead ECG machine, arterial line setup, cardiac monitor, crash cart with defibrillator/pacemaker, manual resuscitation device, oral airway, simulated medications, identification band for patient, role name tags for team members, clipboard with ICU flow sheet, lab results, 12-lead ECG results, physician's orders, telephone, code blue button, albumin, and blood tubing, IV pumps, D_5W, and blue pads.
Introduction	**Administer pre-test** This is day 3 in ICU for patient with liver failure.
Body of scenario	Patient progresses from liver failure to experiencing complications of severe liver failure including respiratory distress, changes in mentation, and renal failure. Lab values show a marked deterioration from the beginning of the scenario to the end.
Conclusion	Patient is being prepared to be intubated and ventilated, family members are at bedside, and a family conference is planned.
Debriefing	**Administer post-test**

Critical Care Simulation

Liver Failure Case 7.0

Scenario number: 7.0 **Scenario focus:** Chronic liver failure/hepatic encephalopathy **Scenario level:** Critical care **Admission type:** ICU **Patient name:** Daniel Arthur Adams **Unique number:** 1786800 **Case number:** 7.0 **Date of birth:** June 1, 1957 **Age:** 54 **Gender:** Male **Attending:** Gina Hawkins, MD **Scenario start day:** Monday **Scenario start time:** 0700 **Admitting diagnosis:** Chronic liver failure **Primary diagnosis:** Chronic liver failure **Secondary diagnosis:** Depression, alcoholism. **Recommended scenario time limit:** 20–25 minutes **Recommended debriefing time limit:** 20–30 minutes	**Scenario purpose:** Nursing management of the patient experiencing liver failure in a critical care practice setting **Learning objectives:** The student will 1. Perform a focused assessment based on the patient's complaint or change in the patient's status. 2. Recognize normal and abnormal assessment findings. 3. Recognize abnormal lab values related to liver failure. 4. Prioritize interventions based on findings and assessments. 5. Document assessment findings. 6. Recognize and manage complications associated with liver failure. 7. Discuss rationales for medications and diagnostics ordered for the patient experiencing liver failure. 8. Recognize signs of respiratory distress and impending respiratory failure and intervene appropriately. 9. Demonstrate ability to analyze dysrhythmias and intervene appropriately. **Learning resources:** Reading assignment: Morton, P., & Fontaine, D. (2009). *Critical care nursing: A holistic approach* (9th ed., Chapter 41). Philadelphia: Lippincott Williams & Wilkins. Susla, G., Suffredini, A., McAreavey, D., Solomom, M., Hoffman, D., & Nyquist, P. (2006). *The handbook of critical care drug therapy* (3rd ed.). Philadelphia: Lippincott Williams & Wilkins. **Simulation Student Workbook activities:** Chronic Liver Failure Case 7.0 in student workbook. Student to complete pre-simulation.

RN to RN Handoff Report

Mr. Adams is a 54-year-old patient admitted to ICU 3 days ago. He has a 10-year history of chronic liver failure and was brought to emergency initially by his family. On admission, he was disoriented and was experiencing loss of appetite, diarrhea, nausea, and vomiting. He has a 15-year history of alcoholism and has attended treatment programs on two occasions with the last being 4 months ago. Mr. Adams also suffers from depression and recently was laid off from his full-time job at an automotive company.

Currently: Heart rate 94 (sinus rhythm with premature ventricular contractions), blood pressure 92/60 mm Hg, respiratory rate 22, temperature 36.4°C, SaO$_2$ 95%, on FiO$_2$ 0.40 by face mask

He has been disoriented and has a markedly distended abdomen, scleral icterus, muscle weakness and tenderness, and palmar erythema.

Right radial arterial line

Triple-lumen central line transduced catheter with D$_5$W infusing at 50 mL/hr through each of the two ports with the third port transduced port

Foley catheter draining small amount of light-brown urine

His blood work results and physician's orders are attached

SaO$_2$, blood oxygen saturation; FiO$_2$, fraction of inspired oxygen.

Simulation Scenario Introduction

Situation/Transition	Facilitator Action	Expected Student Behavioral Outcomes	Resources
Orientation	1. Describe the setting 2. Describe simulation experience 3. Review simulator function (if needed)		• Simulator Directions for simulator manual

Pre-test (optional)	4. Administer pre-test
	  a. Online quiz
	    or
	  b. Response system (i.e., I-clickers)
			• Pre-simulation quiz attached
			• I-clicker questions

Report (see instructor script)	5. Provide report by one of the following options:
	  a. Audio
	  b. Video
	  c. Script (instructor read)
	  d. Script (student read)
		1. Student will make notes based on key points of report.	• View RN to RN handoff report
			• Smart phone download (audio and/or video)
			• Video

Start simulation	1. Select scenario 7.0 program file 2. Start simulation program		• Simulator Directions for simulator manual
Phase I Introduction			
Physiologic state: Currently: HR 94 (sinus rhythm with PVCs), BP 92/60, RR 22, temperature 36.4°C, SaO$_2$ 95% on FiO$_2$ 0.40 by face mask. CVP 15 Patient has been disoriented and has a markedly distended abdomen, scleral icterus, muscle weakness and tenderness, and palmar erythema. Patient states his "legs feel really tired"	3. Progress patient situation Overview Recipe Card 7.0 4. Select "Phase II Body of Scenario" from simulation software menu within 5 minutes *Recommended time to advance: 5 minutes*	1. Student will perform a focused assessment based on the patient's complaint or change in the patient's status. 2. Student will recognize normal and abnormal assessment findings. 3. Student will recognize abnormal lab values related to liver failure. 4. Student will prioritize interventions based on findings and assessments. 5. Student will document assessment findings.	• Overview Recipe Card 7.0

(Continued)

Situation/Transition	Facilitator Action	Expected Student Behavioral Outcomes	Resources
Phase II Body of Scenario			
Physiologic state: (3 hours later) Patient's condition worsens; he begins to develop respiratory distress RR 26 breaths/min SaO$_2$ 91% Patient states he is very short of breath. Crackles now heard in lung bases HR 114 bpm (sinus tachycardia with increasing PVCs) BP 80/40 mm Hg No urine output in the last hour Patient not responding verbally, just moaning incoherently Family members come to bedside (optional, depending on roles and number in group)	5. Progress patient situation following Overview Recipe Card 7.0 6. Select "Phase II Conclusion" from simulation software menu within 10 minutes *Recommended time to advance:* 5–10 minutes Provide student with new ABG results	1. Student will recognize and manage complications associated with liver failure. 2. Student will discuss rationale for medications and diagnostics ordered for the patient experiencing acute liver failure. 3. Student will recognize signs of respiratory distress and impending respiratory failure and intervene appropriately. 4. Student will demonstrate ability to analyze dysrhythmias and intervene appropriately. 5. Student will manage low BP with inotropes and fluids as ordered. 6. Student will contact/notify the physician of patient's respiratory distress, lack of urine output, increasing levels of ammonia, and significant change in level of consciousness.	• Overview Recipe Card 7.0
Phase III Conclusion			
Physiologic state: Patient is in severe respiratory ... PVCs ... ...es ... ...ives and decides to intubate and ventilate the patient Family conference is conducted at bedside with patient's son, physician, and RN End simulation	7. End scenario 8. Save debriefing log	1. Student will demonstrate advanced communication skills with family, physician, and the patient in an emergency situation. 2. Student will assist the physician with intubation. 3. Student participates in family conference using advanced communication skills. 4. Student will demonstrate ability to provide a concise, thorough hand-off report to the oncoming shift.	• Simulator Directions for simulator manual • Simulator Directions for simulator manual

HR, heart rate; PVC, premature ventricular contraction; BP, blood pressure; RR, respiratory rate; SaO$_2$, blood oxygen saturation; FiO$_2$, fraction of inspired oxygen; CVP, central venous pressure; ABG, arterial blood gas; pCO$_2$, partial press of carbon dioxide; HCO$_3$, bicarbonate; pO$_2$, partial pressure of oxygen.

Simulation Follow-up

Situation/Transition	Instructor Action	Expected Student Behavioral Outcomes	Resources
Debriefing	1. Allow students to discuss experience 2. Discuss student performance 3. Watch video of simulation (optional) 4. Administer post-test 5. Online quiz 6. Response system 7. Administer post-simulation survey (optional) 8. Instruct students to complete self-evaluation/reflection (optional) 9. Provide remediation, if needed	1. Student demonstrates ability to reflect on the scenario and discusses actions that were appropriate and interventions to modify for next time. 2. Student completes post-test.	• Debriefing/reflection guide • Post-simulation quiz • I-clicker questions • Textbook: Morton, P., & Fontaine, D. (2009). *Critical care nursing: A holistic approach* (9th ed., Chapter 41). Philadelphia: Lippincott Williams & Wilkins. • Simulation Student Workbook: Chronic liver failure follow-up questions.

Lab Results

Patient Identification
Daniel Arthur Adams
Unique number: 1786800

Test	Result	Normal Ranges
Chemistry Panel:		
Sodium	130	135–1425 mEq/L
Chloride	101	98–107 mEq/L
Potassium	4.8	3.5–5.1 mEq/L
Magnesium	1.1	1.3–2.1 mEq/L
BUN	7.1	6–20 mg/dL (Elderly >60 years old: 8–23 mg/dL)
Creatinine	118	0.4–1.3 mg/dL
Carbon dioxide, total		22–30 mEq/L
Glucose	115	62–110 mg/dL
Lactate		5–20 mg/dL
Calcium		8.6–10.3 mg/dL
Ionized calcium		4.8–5.2
Phosphorus	2.2	2.4–5.1
HbA1C		4.0–6.7% (of total hemoglobin H)
BNP		<100 pg/mL (or <100 ng/L)
CBC:		
WBC	12.1	$4.5–11.0 \times 10^3$
RBC	4.76	Men: $4.6–6.2 \times 10^6$ Women: $4.2–5.4 \times 10^6$
Hgb	13.8	Men: 14.0–17.4 g/dL Women: 12.0–16.0 g/dL
Hct	49	Men: 42–52% Women: 37–47%
Platelets	200	$150–300 \times 10^3$

BUN, blood urea nitrogen; CBC, complete blood count; WBC, white blood cells; RBC, red blood cells; Hgb, hemoglobin.

Test	Result	Normal Ranges
PT	10	12–14 seconds
PTT		18–28 seconds
INR		0.8–1.2
ALT	310	7–56 U/L
ALP	188	38– 26 U/L
Amylase	42	30–110 U/L
AST	350	<35 u/l
Ammonia	72	15–45 mcg/dL
Troponin I		<0.03 ng/mL
Serum albumin	2.5	3.5–5.2 g/dL
Arterial Blood Gases:		
Blood pH	7.33	7.34–7.44
HCO₃	24	22–26 mEq/L
pCO₂	51	35–45 mm Hg
pO₂	78	75 –100

PT, prothrombin time; INR, international normalized ratio; ALT, alanine transaminase; ALP, alkaline phosphatase; AST, aspartate aminotransferase.

Hospital File

Simulation Hospital

Physician's Order Record

Daniel Arthur Adams
Unique Patient Number: 1786800

1. Use ballpoint pen.
2. Draw a line through orders not required and initial.

Admitting diagnosis: Liver failure Allergies: NKDA	Code Status: Full code

Monitoring:
- ✓ Record VS q15 min until stable then q1h
- ✓ Continuous cardiac monitoring
- ✓ CVP q1h
- ✓ Pulmonary capillary occlusive pressure q1h
- ✓ Cardiac output/cardiac index/SVR q4h

Activity:
- ✓ Bed rest
- ✓ Position patient supine with HOB raised 30 degrees
  *keep HOB raised >30 degrees when possible

Diet:
- ☐ NPO
- ☐ Heart smart
- ☐ 1800 kcal diabetic diet
- ✓ Enteral feedings: Insert small-bore feeding tube and commence feeds.
  Type_____Rate_____
- ✓ Consult dietician
- ✓ Sodium and fluid restriction (input = output)
- ✓ Restricted protein diet

(Continued)

IV:

Total fluid to infuse_____ 100 _____ hourly
- ✓ D_5W at 75 mL/hr via side port
- ☐ Lactated Ringer's at_____ /hr
- ✓ D_5W at 25 mL/hr via RA port
- ☐ Other:_____
- ✓ Hemodynamic lines to maintain patency with NS under pressure

O_2:

Titrate O_2 to maintain SaO_2 >95%
If mechanically ventilated:
ETT inserted by_____ at_____ cm

Mode:

_____ SIMV_____ Assist Control_____ Pressure Support_____ Pressure Control_____ CPAP
Rate:_____ Tidal volume_____
FiO_2_____ PEEP_____
- ☐ Withhold sedation at 0600 for assessment of weaning

Medications:
- ☐ Aspirin, enteric coated_____ mg PO daily
- ☐ Acetaminophen 650 mg PO q6h PRN for pain or temperature >38.5°C
- ☐ Ceftazidime 500 mg IV q8h
- ☐ Cefazolin 1g IV q8h
- ☐ Dalteparin 5000 units SQ daily
- ☐ Furosemide_____ mg IV daily
- ☐ Fentanyl_____ mcg q1h PRN
- ☐ Heparin 5000 units SQ q12h
- ☐ Hydromorphone 0.5–1.0 mg IV q1h PRN
- ☐ Metoprolol_____ PO/ng_____
- ☐ Midazolam 2–4 mg IV q1–2h PRN
- ✓ Morphine 2–4 mg IV q1–2h PRN
- ☐ Ondansetron 4 mg q_____ h PRN
- ☐ Insulin Protocol

capillary blood glucose q2h
Goal 80 to 110 mg/dL
Blood glucose = Units/hour
Less than 70 = off
70–89 = 0.2 unit/hour
90–99 = 0.5 unit/hour
100–129 = 1 unit/hour
130–179 = 1.5 unit/hour
180–239 = 2 unit/hour
240–299 = 3 unit/hour
300–359 = 4 unit/hour
>20 notify physician
- ☐ Vancomycin_____ g q_____ h IV

Infusions:
- ☐ Voluven_____ mL if urine output <0.5 mL/kg/hr or CVP <_____
- ☐ Nitroglycerin 100 mg/250 mL D_5W at_____ mcg/hr to maximum_____.
  Titrate for chest pain
- ✓ Dopamine 400 mg/250 mL D_5W start at mcg/kg/min titrate to maintain systolic BP >90
- ☐ Epinephrine 2 mg/250 mL NS at_____ to_____ mcg/min to maintain_____ >_____
- ☐ Dobutamine 250 mg/250 mL NS or D_5W at_____ to_____ to maintain_____ >_____
- ☐ Norepinephrine 4 mg/250 mL D_5W at_____ to_____ maintain_____
- ☐ Vasopressin 20 U/hr_____ to_____ to maintain_____ >_____

(Continued)

✓ Other:
✓ Lactulose 30 mL QID via NG tube
✓ Ranitidine 50 mg IV q8h
✓ Albumin 5% × 1
✓ Neomycin 1 g via NG tube q4h × 24 hr.
✓ Solumedrol 40 mg IV daily
✓ Vitamin B_{12} 30 mcg IM daily × 5
✓ Folic acid 0.4 mg via NG daily

Chest pain protocol:
If chest pain occurs, obtain stat ECG.
✓ Nitroglycerin 0.4 mg spray SL PRN for chest pain. May repeat q5min × 2 (maximum
    3 doses). Then notify the physician.

12-lead ECG on arrival
✓ Repeat ECG daily

Lab tests:
✓ Albumin daily
✓ Bilirubin daily
✓ CBC daily
✓ Chemistry daily (electrolytes, glucose, urea, creatinine)
☐ Cardiac enzymes and troponin q8h × 3
☐ Cross and type_____ units
✓ ABG daily and PRN
☐ Calcium daily
☐ Magnesium daily
✓ PTT/PT/INR daily
✓ If patient becomes febrile, obtain blood cultures × 2
✓ ALT, AST, alkaline phosphatase, BUN, creatinine, ammonia q12h

Diagnostic tests:
✓ Chest x-ray (portable) daily
☐ Echo
☐ Ultrasound_____
✓ MRI liver
✓ Liver biopsy to be done in a.m.

Treatments:
✓ Daily weights
✓ Delirium score BID
☐ Change dressing as per protocol
✓ Physiotherapy

Other:
✓ Arterial line
✓ PA catheter
✓ Foley catheter to hourly output

Physician's Signature:_____ Date_____ Time_____
Nurse's Signature:_____ Date_____ Time_____

Pre- and Post-test Questions

Pre-test Questions	Expected Answer/Reference
1. What complications can arise as a result of liver failure?	Infection Hemorrhage Renal failure Respiratory failure Acid–base imbalances Fluid and electrolyte disturbances Hepatic encephalopathy and coma Morton, P., & Fontaine, D. (2009). *Critical care nursing: A holistic approach* (9th ed., Chapter 41, pp. 1073–1074). Philadelphia: Lippincott Williams & Wilkins.
2. What lab work is essential to monitor for the patient with liver failure?	ALT, AST, alkaline phosphatase, bilirubin, GGT, albumin, glucose, BUN, creatinine, ammonia, electrolytes, Hgb, INR, and PT Morton, P., & Fontaine, D. (2009). *Critical care nursing: A holistic approach* (9th ed., Chapter 41, p. 1075). Philadelphia: Lippincott Williams & Wilkins. Diepenbrock, N. (2012). *Quick reference to critical care* (4th ed., p. 232). Philadelphia: Lippincott Williams & Wilkins.
3. What are some of the causes of liver failure?	Acetaminophen overdose, long-term alcohol ingestion, chronic viral hepatitis, prolonged cholestasis, and metabolic disorders Morton, P., & Fontaine, D. (2009). *Critical care nursing: A holistic approach* (9th ed., Chapter 41, p. 1073). Philadelphia: Lippincott Williams & Wilkins.

Post-test Questions	Expected Answer/Reference
1. What was the significance of the rising serum ammonia level?	Increases are due to the liver's failing ability to clear nitrogenous and other waste products. Increased ammonia levels cause hepatic encephalopathy because of toxic effects on the brain tissue. Morton, P., & Fontaine, D. (2009). *Critical care nursing: A holistic approach* (9th ed., Chapter 41, p. 1078–1079). Philadelphia: Lippincott Williams & Wilkins.
2. What was the significance and purpose of lactulose being ordered for this patient?	Lactulose decreases the pH in the colon and helps cause migration of ammonia from the blood to the colon where it can be excreted, thereby lowering ammonia levels in the blood. Morton, P., & Fontaine, D. (2009). *Critical care nursing: A holistic approach* (9th ed., Chapter 41, p. 1079). Philadelphia: Lippincott Williams & Wilkins.
3. What were the "red flags" or signs that the patient was worsening?	Lab values (i.e., ammonia levels) continue to worsen instead of returning to normal levels The presence of respiratory distress, onset of renal failure, dysrhythmias, altered and obtunded mentation, hemorrhage, and infection. Morton, P., & Fontaine, D. (2009). *Critical care nursing: A holistic approach* (9th ed., Chapter 41, pp. 1075, 1079). Philadelphia: Lippincott Williams & Wilkins.

ALT, alanine aminotransferase; AST, aspartate aminotransferase; GGT, gamma-glutamyl transpeptidase; BUN, blood urea nitrogen; Hgb, hemoglobin; INR, international normalized ratio; PT, prothrombin time.

Competency Checklist

Liver Failure Case 7.0

Name: **Date:**

Competency	Examples	Met	Unmet	Comments
Performs appropriate assessment	Comprehensive			
12- and 15-lead ECG proficiency	Performs 12-lead ECG 12-lead ECG interpretation Performs 15-lead ECG			
Demonstrates ability to correctly interpret arrhythmia	• Sinus rhythm with PVCs • Sinus tachycardia • Ventricular tachycardia			
Demonstrates safe management of hemodynamic monitoring	Triple-lumen central line CVP Arterial catheter			
Demonstrates safe management of oxygenation	Ventilation modes Arterial blood gas interpretation Troubleshoots ventilator alarms			
Demonstrates safe administration of pharmacological agents	Morphine Dopamine infusion Regular insulin Ranitidine			
Accurately interprets lab values	Chemistry Hematology Arterial blood gases			
Demonstrates ability to quickly recognize and prioritize a patient's rapidly deteriorating condition	Hypotension Decreased level of consciousness Assessment of respiratory distress Notes presence of respiratory crackles			
Demonstrates principles related to safe patient care	Alarms on Accurate hand-off report Communication with patient and 　health care team Lines secured Independent double checks Positioning			
Specific	Communication with family/family 　conference Able to suggest anticipated ventilator 　changes based on ABGs and 　changing patient condition Suctions ETT as appropriate Follows best practice guidelines for 　VAP prevention			

Feedback: _____
_____
_____
_____

Instructor: _____

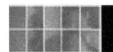

Trauma Case 8.0

Overview Recipe Card

Patient: Vijay Surendra

Scenario 8.0

Learning objectives	The student will
	1. Perform a focused assessment based on the patient's complaint or change in the patient's status. 2. Recognize normal and abnormal assessment findings. 3. Prioritize interventions based on findings and assessments. 4. Document assessment findings. 5. Demonstrate ability to manage chest drainage systems. 6. Demonstrate ability to identify and prevent complications from multiple system traumas. 7. Demonstrate ability to manage the technology/patient interface. 8. Administer medications accurately and identify indications, contraindications, and side effects associated with interventions. 9. Call for team assistance as appropriate and manage a patient experiencing hypoxemia. 10. Initiate primary ABC measures and safely manage hypoxemia. 11. Demonstrate ability to provide a concise, thorough hand-off report to the oncoming shift.
Equipment needed	12-lead ECG machine, arterial line and central venous pressure monitor to 500 mL pressurized normal saline solution, triple lumen catheter, 1000 mL lactated Ringer's solution, 250 mL normal saline solution, × 2 infusion pumps, chest tube with drainage system connected to wall suction, manual resuscitation device, oral suction, #7 endotracheal tube with ties or tape for securing, ventilator, cardiac monitor, crash cart with defibrillator/pacemaker and intubation tray, face mask with flow meter, simulated medications, blood collection tubes (for ABG, complete cell count, and electrolyte analyses), Vacutainer holder, identification band for patient, role name tags for team members, clip board with ICU flow sheet, lab results, 12-lead ECG results and physician's orders, telephone, code blue button. Also, * dressing for left thigh, cast material for left arm, occlusive dressing for left chest wall over chest tube * diaphoresis mode on simulator or spray bottle for moisture on forehead * cyanosis of fingertips mode on simulator
Introduction	**Administer pre-test.**
Body of scenario	The day after admission to the ICU, the multisystem trauma patient (fractured left ribs, left radius/ulna, and left femur) becomes short of breath and restless, while his SaO$_2$ level drops. Patient requires intubation and mechanical ventilation.
Conclusion	Patient is intubated, mechanically ventilated, and sedated. Family members are present.
Debriefing	**Administer post-test.**

Critical Care Simulation

Trauma Case 8.0

Scenario number: 8.0 **Scenario focus:** Trauma **Scenario level:** Critical care **Admission type:** ICU **Patient name:** Vijay Surendra **Unique number:** 1786812 **Case number:** 8.0 **Date of birth:** November 20, 1987 **Age:** 24 **Gender:** M **Attending:** Nathan Burke, MD **Scenario start day:** Tuesday **Scenario start time:** 0700 **Admitting diagnosis:** Trauma **Primary diagnosis:** Fractured ribs left side 5–9, pulmonary contusions, fractured left radius and ulna, fractured left femur, fractured pelvis **Secondary diagnosis:** **Recommended scenario time limit:** 20–25 minutes **Recommended debriefing time limit:** 20–30 minutes	**Scenario purpose:** Nursing management of the patient experiencing multiple trauma and subsequent hypoxemia resulting from fat emboli, in a critical care practice setting. **Learning objectives:** The student will 1. Perform a focused assessment based on the patient's complaint or change in the patient's status. 2. Recognize normal and abnormal assessment findings. 3. Prioritize interventions based on findings and assessments. 4. Document assessment findings. 5. Demonstrate ability to manage chest drainage systems. 6. Demonstrate ability to identify and prevent complications from multiple system trauma. 7. Demonstrate ability to manage the technology/patient interface. 8. Administer medications accurately and identify indications, contraindications, and side effects associated with interventions. 9. Call for team assistance as appropriate including management of a patient experiencing hypoxemia. 10. Initiate primary ABC measures and safely manage hypoxemia. 11. Demonstrate ability to provide a concise, thorough, hand-off report to the oncoming shift. **Learning resources:** Reading assignment: 1. Morton, P., & Fontaine, D. (2009). *Critical care nursing: A holistic approach* (9th ed., pp. 1437–1453). Philadelphia: Lippincott Williams & Wilkins. 2. Diepenbrock, N. (2012). *Quick reference to critical care* (4th ed., pp. 382–383). Philadelphia: Lippincott Williams & Wilkins. 3. Bickley, L., & Szilagyi, P. (2009). *Bates guide to physical examination and history taking* (10th ed., pp. 296–309, 591–637). Philadelphia: Lippincott Williams & Wilkins. 4. Diehl, T. (editor). *Critical care made incredibly easy.* (2004) (p. 644). Philadelphia: Lippincott Williams & Wilkins. **Simulation Student Workbook activities:** Trauma 8.0 in student workbook. Student to complete pre-simulation.

RN to RN Handoff Report

Vijay Surendra is a 24-year-old male patient of Dr. Burke. He was admitted the day before after sustaining multiple injuries in a motor vehicle crash. While driving along a country road alone, he was hit on the driver's side by another car that was proceeding through a stop sign. Vijay's cervical spine x-rays were cleared in the ER by Dr. Mark. After fluid resuscitation, it was noted that Vijay sustained fractured ribs, left side ribs 5–9 with pulmonary contusions, fractured left radius and ulna, fractured left femur, and fractured pelvis. A #32 chest tube was inserted at the fifth intercostal space, midclavicular line, and connected to a chest tube drainage system with 20 cm suction. The system drained a moderate amount of sanguineous matter. Vijay was stabilized in the ER, taken to the OR for an open reduction and internal fixation of the left femur, and returned to the CCU. Left ulnar and radial fractures were stabilized with a cast. Pelvic fracture was stable. Distal circulation to all limbs was satisfactory, although petechiae are noted over the chest. A triple-lumen catheter was placed in the right internal jugular vein. A right radial arterial line, nasogastric tube (via the right nare), and a Foley catheter were placed in the ER. Over the past 24 hours, Vijay has been stable. Vijay's family has been notified by the authorities.

BP 96/55 mm Hg, HR 120 bpm, RR 29 breaths/min, SaO_2 94%, temperature 37.8°C, urine output 50 mL/hr.

No past surgeries or health concerns. Patient smokes cigarettes, a pack per day.

He has no known allergies.

His blood work results and physician's orders are attached.

ER, emergency room; OR, operating room; CCU, critical care unit.

Simulation Scenario

Situation/Transition	Facilitator Action	Expected Student Behavioral Outcomes	Resources
Orientation	1. Describe the setting 2. Describe simulation experience 3. Review simulator function (if needed)		• Simulator Directions for simulator manual

Pre-test (optional)	4. Administer pre-test
	  a. Online quiz
	    or
	  b. Response system (i.e., I-clickers)
			• Pre-simulation quiz attached
			• I-clicker questions

Report (see instructor script)	5. Provide report by one of the following options:
	  a. Audio
	  b. Video
	  c. Script (instructor read)
	  d. Script (student read).
		1. Student will make notes based on key points of report.	• View RN to RN Handoff Report
			• Smart phone download (audio and/or video)
			• Video

Start simulation	1. Select Scenario 8.0 program file. 2. Start simulation program. Set up vital signs and beginning of patient parameters.		• Simulator Directions for simulator manual
Phase I Introduction			
Physiologic state: HR 120 bpm (sinus tachycardia) BP 96/55 mm Hg via right radial arterial line RR 28 breaths/min CVP 12 mm Hg Temperature 37.8°C SaO_2 94% on FiO_2 at. 0.50 by face mask Breath sounds clear, decreased to bases Urinary output 50 mL, straw-colored urine Lactated Ringer's solution at 125 mL/hr via distal port, normal saline solution at 25 mL/hr via medial port, and distal port is transduced for CVP monitoring	3. Progress patient's situation following Overview Recipe Card 8.0 *Recommended time to advance scenario:* 10 minutes	1. Student conducts systematic patient assessment and correctly assesses chest drainage system. 2. Student checks orders and lab values, and calculates IV drip rates for accuracy, verbalizes understanding of medications, indications, and side effects parameters to assess. 3. Student assesses all hemodynamic lines, waveforms, and values and demonstrates correct method for zeroing, leveling, and calibrating equipment. 4. Student compares cuff blood pressure to intra-arterial pressure. 5. Student analyzes cardiac rhythm accurately. 6. Student uses advanced communication strategies for communicating with the anxious patient, the patient's family (if present), and other members of the health care team. 7. Student documents accurately on ICU flow sheet. 8. Student demonstrates ability to accurately interpret lab results and recognizes abnormal values.	• Overview Recipe Card 8.0

(Continued)

Situation/Transition	Facilitator Action	Expected Student Behavioral Outcomes	Resources
Phase II Body of Scenario			
Physiologic state: Monitor begins to alarm patient as SaO$_2$ deteriorates from 94% to 85%. Patient becomes restless and anxious. *Diaphoretic and cyanotic fingertips HR 140 bpm (sinus tachycardia with ST segment elevation) Blood pressure 90/40 mm Hg RR 38 breaths/min CVP 14 mm Hg Breath sounds: crackles throughout both lung fields Urinary output 50 mL straw-colored urine Patient says, "I can't breathe. Help."	4. Progress patient's situation following Overview Recipe Card 8.0. 5. Select "Phase II Outcome" from simulation software menu within 10 minutes. *Recommended time to advance scenario:* 5 minutes. Provides student with "stat lab results"	1. Student demonstrates ability to recognize deterioration in condition and calls physician stat. 2. Student notes decreased SaO$_2$ and patient's instability and immediately calls for help. 3. Student attempts maneuvers to increase SaO$_2$. 4. Student sends blood to lab for stat analysis of ABGs, CBC, and electrolyte. 5. When physician or RT arrives, student assists with intubation and mechanical ventilation. 6. Once the patient is stabilized, student verbalizes need for chest x-ray, ECG, and ABG analysis are performed. 7. In collaboration with team, student suggests potential causes for abrupt deterioration.	• Overview Recipe Card 8.0
Phase III Conclusion of Scenario			
Physiologic state: Patient is sedated. HR 110 bpm (sinus tachycardia with ST segment elevation) BP 95/40 mm Hg RR 18 breaths/min SaO$_2$ 98% CVP 14 mm Hg Urinary output 50 mL straw-colored urine Mechanically ventilated: SIMV rate 12; tidal volume 500 mL; FiO$_2$ 0.60; PEEP 5 cm *End Simulation*		1. Student performs a focused respiratory reassessment. 2. Student provides update to family.	Prepare to go to debriefing session.

HR, heart rate; BP, blood pressure; RR, respiratory rate; CVP, central venous pressure; SIMV, synchronized intermittent mandatory ventilation; PEEP, positive end-expiratory pressure; ABGs, arterial blood gases; SaO$_2$, blood oxygen saturation; FiO$_2$, fraction of inspired oxygen; RT, respiratory therapist.

Simulation Follow-up

Situation/Transition	Instructor Action	Expected Student Behavioral Outcomes	Resources
Debriefing	1. Allow students to discuss experience. 2. Discuss student performance. 3. Watch video of simulation (optional). 4. Administer post-test (attached) a. Online quiz b. Response system. 5. Administer post-simulation survey (optional). 6. Instruct students to complete self-evaluation/reflection (optional). 7. Provide remediation, if needed.	1. Student demonstrates ability to reflect on the scenario and discusses actions that were appropriate and interventions to modify for next time. 2. Student completes post-test.	• I-clicker questions • Post-test • Simulation Student Workbook follow-up assignment.

Lab Results (Scene 1)

Patient Identification
Vijay Surendra
Unique number: 1786812

Test	Result	Normal Ranges
Chemistry Panel:		
Sodium	132	135–1425 mEq/L
Chloride	101	98–107 mEq/L
Potassium	3.9	3.5–5.1 mEq/L
Magnesium		1.3–2.1 mEq/L
BUN	7.2	6–20 mg/dL (Elderly >60 years old: 8–23 mg/dL)
Creatinine	0.75	0.4–1.3 mg/dL
Carbon dioxide, total		22–30 mEq/L
Glucose	73	62–110 mg/dL
Lactate		5–20 mg/dL
Calcium		8.6–10.3 mg/dL
Ionized calcium		4.8–5.2
Phosphorus		2.4–5.1
HbA1C		4.0–6.7% (of total hemoglobin H)
BNP		<100 pg/mL (or <100 ng/L)
CBC:		
WBC	18	4.5–11.0 × 10^3
RBC	3.48	Men: 4.6–6.2 × 10 ϖ Women: 4.2–5.4 × 10 ϖ
Hgb	9.4	Men: 14.0–17.4 g/dL Women: 12.0–16.0 g/dL
Hct	41	Men: 42–52% Women: 37–47%
Platelets	98	150–300 × 10^3

Test	Result	Normal Ranges
PT	12	12–14 seconds
PTT	22	18–28 seconds
INR		0.8–1.2
Liver enzymes:		
ALT		7–56 U/L
ALP		38–126 U/L
Amylase		30–110 U/L
Troponin I		<0.03 ng/mL
Serum lactate		5–20 mg/dL
Arterial Blood Gases:		
Blood pH	7.35	7.34–7.44
HCO_3	23	22–26 mEq/L
pCO_2	45	35–45 mm Hg
pO_2	83	75–100 mm Hg

PT, prothrombin time; PTT, partial thromboplastin time; INR, international normalized ratio; ALT, alanine transaminase; ALP, alkaline phosphatase.

Stat Lab Results

Date/Time:_____ Patient Name:_____ Vijay Surendra_____

Hematology	**Chemistry**
Hgb:_____Hct:_____	Na: 133 K: 4.5
WBC:_____Platelets:_____	Cl: 110 HCO_3: 22
Other:	Urea: 21 Creatinine: 390
	Glucose:_____
	CPK:_____Troponin:_____
	AST:_____ALT:
	Other:
	ABGs:
	pH 7.33, PCO_2 50, PO_2 55, HCO_3 22
Coagulation Studies	**Urinalysis**
PT:_____PTT:_____	pH:_____
INR:_____	Glucose:_____
Bleeding time:_____	Ketones:_____
D-Dimers:_____	Specific gravity:_____
Fibrin split products:_____	Blood:_____
Other:	Protein:_____
	Leukocyte:_____

Hgb, hemoglobin; WBC, white blood cells; CPK, creatine phosphokinase; ABGs, arterial blood gases.

Simulation Hospital

Physician's Order Record

Patient Identification
Vijay Surendra
Unique number: 1786812

1. Use ballpoint pen.
2. Draw a line through orders not required and initial.

Admitting diagnosis: MVC Trauma #left ribs 5, 6, 7, 8, and 9; pulmonary contusions, #left radius and ulna, #left femur April 4, 2011. Operating room (OR)-open reduction and internal fixation left femur Allergies: none Monitoring: ✓ Record VS q15 min until stable then q1h ✓ Continuous cardiac monitoring ✓ CVP q1h ☐ Pulmonary artery occlusive pressure q_____h ☐ Cardiac output/cardiac index/SVR q_____h	Code Status: Full

Activity:
 ✓ Bed rest
 ✓ Position supine with HOB raised <u>30</u> degrees
  *keep HOB raised more than 30 degrees when possible

Diet:
 ✓ NPO
 ☐ Heart smart
 ☐ 1800 kcal diabetic diet
 ☐ Enteral feeds: insert small-bore feeding tube and commence feedings.
Type_____rate_____
 ✓ Consult dietitian regarding nutrition

IV:
Total fluid to infuse <u>150 mL</u> hourly
 ✓ NS at <u>25 mL/h</u>
 ✓ Lactated Ringer's at <u>125 mL/hr</u>
 ☐ D_5W at_____/hr
 ☐ Other:_____
 ✓ Hemodynamic lines to maintain patency with NS under pressure

O_2:
Titrate O_2 to maintain SaO_2 ><u>95</u>%
If mechanically ventilated:
ETT inserted by_____at_____cm
Mode:
_____SIMV_____Assist Control_____Pressure Support_____Pressure
Control_____CPAP
Rate:_____Tidal volume_____
FiO_2_____PEEP_____
 ☐ Withhold sedation at 0600 for assessment of weaning

(Continued)

Medications:
- ☐ Aspirin, enteric coated_____mg PO daily
- ✓ Acetaminophen 650 mg PO q6h PRN for pain or temperature >38.5°C
- ☐ Ceftazidime 500 mg IV q8h
- ✓ Cefazolin 1 g IV Q8h
- ☐ Dalteparin 5000 units SQ daily
- ☐ Furosemide_____mg IV daily
- ☐ Fentanyl_____mcg q1h PRN
- ✓ Heparin 5000 units SQ q12h <u>reassess in 12 hours</u>
- ☐ Hydromorphone 0.5–1.0 mg IV q1h PRN
- ☐ Metoprolol_____PO/ng_____
- ☐ Midazolam 2–4 mg IV q1–2h PRN
- ✓ Morphine_____IV q1–2h PRN
- ☐ Ondansetron 4 mg q_____h PRN
- ✓ Ranitidine 50 mg IV q8h
- ☐ Insulin Protocol

capillary blood glucose q2h

Goal 80 to 110 mg/dL

Blood glucose = Units/hour

Less than 70 = off

70–89 = 0.2 unit/hour

90–99 = 0.5 unit/hour

100–129 = 1 unit/hour

130–179 = 1.5 unit/hour

180–239 = 2 unit/hour

240–299 = 3 unit/hour

300–359 = 4 unit/hour

>20 notify physician
- ☐ Vancomycin_____g q_____h IV

Infusions:
- ✓ Voluven <u>500</u> mL if urine output less than 0.5 mL/kg/hr or CVP less than_____
- ☐ Nitroglycerin 100 mg/250 mL D_5W at_____mcg/hr to maximum_____.
  Titrate for chest pain
- ✓ Dopamine 200 mg/250 mL D_5W at <u>3</u> to <u>20 mcg/kg/min</u> titrate to
  maintain systolic BP ><u>100 mm</u> Hg
- ☐ Epinephrine 2 mg/250 mL NS at_____to_____mcg/min to
  maintain_____greater than_____
- ☐ Dobutamine 250 mg/250 mL NS or D_5W at_____to_____to
  maintain_____greater than_____
- ☐ Norepinephrine 4 mg/250 mL D_5W at_____to_____maintain_____
- ☐ Vasopressin 20 units/hr_____to_____to maintain_____greater than_____
- ☐ Other:

Chest pain protocol:

If chest pain occurs, obtain stat ECG.
- ☐ Nitroglycerin 0.4 mg spray SL PRN for chest pain. May repeat q5 min ×
  2 (maximum 3 doses). Then notify physician

12-lead ECG on arrival:
- ☐ Repeat ECG q8h ×2
- ✓ Daily ECG

Lab tests:
- ☐ Albumin daily
- ☐ Bilirubin daily
- ✓ CBC daily
- ✓ Chemistry daily (electrolytes, glucose, urea, and creatinine)
- ✓ Cardiac enzymes and troponin q8h ×3
- ✓ Cross and type <u>4</u> units packed red blood cells
- ✓ ABG daily and PRN

(Continued)

☐ Calcium daily ☐ Magnesium daily ☐ PTT/PT daily ✓ If patient becomes febrile, obtain blood for culture × 2 Diagnostic tests: ✓ Chest x-ray (portable) daily ☐ Echo ☐ Ultrasound_____ ☐ CT scan_____	
Treatments: ☐ Daily weights ✓ Delirium score BID ☐ Change dressing as per protocol ✓ Physiotherapy for chest and immobility	
Other: 1. Ortho to follow in the ICU	

Physician's Signature:_____Date_____Time_____
Nurse's Signature:_____Date_____Time_____

Simulation Hospital

Additional Physician's Orders

Date	Intubate and ventilate to maintain pH 7.35–7.45, PCO_2 35–45, PO_2 80–100, SIMV 12/min, tidal volume 500 mL, FiO_2 0.60, PEEP 5 cm Stat portable chest x-ray Stat ABGs, CBC, and electrolytes Signature:	Vijay Surendra 1786812

Pre- and Post-test Questions

Pre-test Questions	Expected Answer/Reference
1. Describe three complications for a patient experiencing a thoracic trauma.	Tracheobronchial trauma (i.e., airway injury, dyspnea, subcutaneous emphysema) Thorax fractures (i.e., rib fractures, sternal fractures, and flail chest) Pleural space injuries (i.e., pneumothorax, hemothorax) Pulmonary contusion (i.e., poor response to increasing FiO_2) Blunt cardiac injury (i.e., dysrhythmias, nonspecific ECG changes) Penetrating cardiac injury (i.e., cardiac tamponade, hypovolemic shock) Cardiac tamponade (i.e., hypovolemic shock, cardiogenic shock) Aortic injury (i.e., aortic rupture, organ ischemia [renal failure, bowel ischemia, lower limb weakness]) Morton, P., & Fontaine, D. (2009). *Critical care nursing: A holistic approach* (9th ed., p. 1417). Philadelphia: Lippincott Williams & Wilkins.

(Continued)

Pre-test Questions	Expected Answer/Reference
2. What is the classic presentation of a cardiac tamponade?	Signs and symptoms of cardiac tamponade: • Beck's triad: decreased BP, muffled heart sounds, and increased central venous pressure • Narrowing pulse pressure • Increased central venous pressure • Widened mediastinum on x-ray film • Cardiac hemodynamic pressures equalizing (e.g., right atrial, pulmonary artery diastolic, pulmonary artery occlusive pressure) • Pulsus paradoxus >10 mm Hg Morton, P., & Fontaine, D. (2009). *Critical care nursing: A holistic approach* (9th ed., p. 1421). Philadelphia: Lippincott Williams & Wilkins. Diepenbrock, N. (2012). *Quick reference to critical care* (4th ed., p. 159). Philadelphia: Lippincott Williams & Wilkins, pp. 51–52.
3. Discuss cultural competence related to critical illness.	Cultural competence involves: • Recognizing the role culture has on a patient's beliefs of health and wellness • Acknowledging one's own ethnocentrism • Recognizing unique cultural, religious, and spiritual practices of each patient and family; do not assume faith and cultural practices are adopted by all • Integrating patient's cultural preferences and alternative healing practices into the plan of care Morton, P., & Fontaine, D. (2009). *Critical care nursing: A holistic approach* (9th ed., p. 40). Philadelphia: Lippincott Williams & Wilkins.

Post-test Questions	Expected Answer/Reference
1. Describe the nursing priority for collaborative management for the patient experiencing multisystem trauma.	Collaborative care with multisystem trauma **Outcome** / **Assessment** / **Intervention** Oxygenation / Assess LOC, airway patency / Auscultate breath sounds. Administer supplemental oxygen. Monitor SaO$_2$ and ABG values. Maintain SaO$_2$ >95%. Perform chest physiotherapy. Manage pain. Intubate/ventilate patient as appropriate. Circulation / Assess for adequate BP, HR, and RR. / Monitor vital signs. Perform continuous cardiac monitoring. Infuse IV fluids/blood products as appropriate. Know the use of vasoactive infusions. Fluids/electrolytes / Determine adequate fluid balance. / Monitor intake and output. Monitor lab values. Mobility and safety / Assess muscle strength to prevent deterioration. / Consult PT/OT regarding the patient's range of motion, mobility, and functions. Encourage early ambulation. Morton, P., & Fontaine, D. (2009). *Critical care nursing: A holistic approach* (9th ed., p. 1416). Philadelphia: Lippincott Williams & Wilkins.

(Continued)

Post-test Questions	Expected Answer/Reference
2. Discuss one complication of musculoskeletal injury for patients experiencing multisystem trauma, relating signs and symptoms, as well as nursing management.	**Compartment syndrome** is a complicating condition that occurs from injury or surgery, where pressure increases within the muscle compartment, compressing arteries, veins, and nerves within and leading to tissue ischemia. In order to save the limb, a fasciotomy is performed. Through careful assessment of the five "P's" and monitoring for a heightened pain response related to the injury, the nurse can intervene by calling the surgeon. **DVT** is a complicating condition in which a thrombus forms in a deep vein, usually in the lower limb, leading to the obstruction of distal blood flow. Through careful assessment, early changes are detected. The use of anticoagulants and compression devices are intended to prevent occurrence of DVT. **Pulmonary embolus,** another complicating condition occurs when a thrombus that has formed in a limb (e.g., the calf) dislodges and travels to the pulmonary vasculature. This life-threatening condition causes dyspnea, chest pain, tachypnea, and hypoxemia. The nurse's role is prevention of clot development by administering DVT prophylaxis as ordered and instructing patient not to cross legs, to begin ambulating as soon as able, to wear compression hose, and so on. **Fat embolism syndrome** occurs after a long bone fracture or a trauma whereby fat globules are released into circulation and lodge in the pulmonary vasculature. The nurse's role is to assess for petechiae over the upper torso and axillae, dyspnea, restlessness, tachycardia, fever, and decreased level of consciousness. Prevention includes minimal handling of fracture prior to surgical intervention, ensuring that the patient is well hydrated, and monitoring SaO_2 and ABGs. Morton, P., & Fontaine, D. (2009). *Critical care nursing: A holistic approach* (9th ed., p. 1430). Philadelphia: Lippincott Williams & Wilkins. Diepenbrock, N. (2012). *Quick reference to critical care* (4th ed., pp. 284, 377). Philadelphia: Lippincott Williams & Wilkins, pp. 51–52.
3. How would the nurse recognize a patient with DIC?	DIC is a secondary condition associated with both hemorrhage and thrombosis. It is triggered by obstetrical conditions (preeclampsia, abruptio placentae), malignant conditions (lymphoma, leukemia, lung cancer), trauma (burns, snakebite, extensive trauma), vascular abnormalities (vasculitis), surgery, immunological disorders (blood transfusion reaction, transplant rejection), infection (gram-negative, gram-positive), acute liver disease. Early stage DIC includes activation of platelets/fibrin leading to circulating thrombi. These thrombi lodge in organs, such as lung, brain, bowel or kidneys, as well as the digits resulting in tissue ischemia. Later, bleeding occurs due to depletion of clotting factors. Bleeding can occur from any surgical site, cannulation site. Intracerebral bleeding, hematuria, hemoptysis, epistaxis, and massive gastrointestinal bleeding can also occur. Lab studies to monitor are platelet counts, prothrombin time, partial thromboplastin time, thrombin time, fibrinogen, fibrin degradation products, and D-Dimer assay. The treatment goal is to detect and remove the underlying cause. The use of heparin therapy is controversial in treating DIC; low molecular weight heparins are often used as an alternative. Clotting factor replacement is administered to stop bleeding or prevent bleeding before an invasive procedure. Monitoring for further bleeding especially from venipuncture sites is necessary and ongoing. Morton, P., & Fontaine, D. (2009). *Critical care nursing: A holistic approach* (9th ed., p. 1303). Philadelphia: Lippincott Williams & Wilkins. Diepenbrock, N. (2012). *Quick reference to critical care* (4th ed., p. 286). Philadelphia: Lippincott Williams & Wilkins.

DVT, deep vein thrombosis; DIC, disseminated intravascular coagulation; LOC, level of consciousness; OT, occupational therapy.

Competency Checklist

Trauma Case 8.0

Name: **Date:**

Competency	Examples	Met	Unmet	Comments
Performs appropriate assessment.	Comprehensive Chest tube Focused respiratory			
Demonstrates ability to correctly interpret arrhythmia and 12-lead ECG.	Sinus tachycardia			
Demonstrates safe management of hemodynamic monitoring.	Arterial line CVP			
Demonstrates safe management of oxygenation.	Ventilation modes Endotracheal tube			
Demonstrates safe administration of pharmacological agents.	Morphine			
Accurately interprets lab values.	Chemistry/Glucose Hematology Urea/Creatinine Arterial blood gases			
Demonstrates ability to quickly recognize and prioritize a patient's rapidly deteriorating condition.	Measures to improve oxygenation Assists with intubation Draws blood for ABGs and electrolytes			
Demonstrates principles related to safe patient care.	Alarms Lines secured Independent double checks Positioning			
Specific:	Establishes patient goal collaboratively Communication with family Identifies cause of hypoxic event			

Feedback:_____

_____

_____

_____

_____

_____

Instructor:_____

Septic Shock Case 9.0

Overview Recipe Card

Patient Name: John French

Scenario 9.0

Learning objectives	The student will 1. Perform a focused assessment based on the patient's complaint or change in the patient's status. 2. Recognize normal and abnormal assessment findings. 3. Identify signs and symptoms of septic shock. 4. Prioritize interventions based on findings and assessments. 5. Document assessment findings. 6. Demonstrate ability to analyze arrhythmias and intervene appropriately. 7. Identify nursing management priorities of a patient in septic shock. 8. Administer medications accurately and identify indications, contraindications, and side effects associated with interventions. 9. Demonstrate ability to accurately calculate vasoactive infusion drips as ordered.
Equipment needed	12-lead ECG machine, arterial line and PA catheter setup, peripheral IV line, cardiac monitor, crash cart with defibrillator/pacemaker, manual resuscitation device and oral airway, simulated medications, identification band for patient, role name tags for team members, clipboard with ICU flow sheet, lab results, 12-lead ECG results and physician's orders, telephone, code blue button, simulated packed RBCs and blood tubing, IV pumps, normal saline solution, fake blood, Foley catheter, abdominal dressing, two Jackson-Pratt drains, and disposable bed pads.
Introduction	**Administer pre-test.** Patient initially admitted to undergo colonoscopy. A perforation of the large bowel occurred during the procedure and the patient subsequently underwent a bowel resection and repair in the OR and was admitted to ICU for observation.
Body of scenario	From day 2 postoperative bowel resection status, the patient's status progresses to developing signs and symptoms of septic shock.
Conclusion	End scenario at a point where the patient requires intubation and ventilation.
Debriefing	**Administer post-test.**

PA, pulmonary artery; RBCs, red blood cells; OR, operating room.

Critical Care Simulation

Septic Shock Case 9.0

<table>
<tr>
<td>

Scenario number: 9.0
Scenario focus: Septic Shock
Scenario level: Critical Care
Admission type: ICU
Patient name: Mr. John French
Unique number: 1786811
Case number: 9.0
Date of birth: December 1, 1965
Age: 46
Gender: M
Attending: Susan Jane Parker, MD
Scenario start day: Wednesday
Scenario start time: 1900
Admitting diagnosis: Rectal bleeding
Primary diagnosis: Perforation of large bowel.
Secondary diagnosis: Bowel resection, sepsis.
Recommended scenario time limit: 20–25 minutes
Recommended debriefing time limit: 20–30 minutes

</td>
<td>

Scenario purpose: Nursing management of the patient experiencing bowel perforation and subsequent septic shock in a critical care practice setting.

Learning objectives:
The student will
1. Perform a focused assessment based on the patient's complaint or change in the patient's status.
2. Recognize normal and abnormal assessment findings.
3. Identify signs and symptoms of septic shock.
4. Prioritize interventions based on findings and assessments.
5. Document assessment findings.
6. Demonstrate ability to analyze dysrhythmias and intervene appropriately.
7. Identify nursing management priorities of a patient in septic shock.
8. Administer medications accurately and identify indications, contraindications, and side effects associated with interventions.
9. Demonstrate ability to accurately calculate IV drip rates for vasoactive drugs as ordered.

Learning resources:
Reading assignment:
1. Morton, P., & Fontaine, D. (2009). In *Critical care nursing: A holistic approach* (9th ed., Chapter 13, pp. 1391–1405). Philadelphia: Lippincott Williams & Wilkins.
2. Susla, G. et al (2006) The handbook of critical care drug therapy (3rd ed.) Philadelphia: Lippincott Williams & Wilkins.

Simulation Student Workbook activities: Septic Shock Case 9.0 in student workbook. Student to complete pre-simulation.

</td>
</tr>
</table>

RN to RN Handoff Report

Mr. French, a 46-year-old male, was admitted to the ICU following colonoscopy and subsequent large bowel perforation. Mr. French suffered a perforated large bowel as a complication to the colonoscopy he underwent Monday morning at 0900. Postcolonoscopy, while in the recovery area, he started to have moderate-to-large sanguineous drainage per rectum. He was taken to the OR where a bowel resection and repair of the perforation to his large bowel was undertaken. Since the OR, he has been hemodynamically unstable and the decision was made to admit him to ICU for observation. He has a history of coronary artery disease and hypertension. He is approximately 100 pounds over his ideal weight. He is currently on FiO_2 0.40 by rebreather mask. He has a large midline abdominal dressing with small amounts of sanguineous drainage, and two Jackson-Pratt drains are draining small amounts of sanguineous fluid.

It is now postoperative day 2 in the ICU.

Mr. French has a right peripheral IV line infusing normal saline solution at 125 mL/hr, a left radial arterial line, a right subclavian pulmonary artery catheter, a nasogastric tube connected to low suction, and a Foley catheter.

His vital signs are as follows:
HR 110 bpm
RR 22 breaths/min
SaO_2 95%
BP 102/64 mm Hg
Temperature 37.4°C
His blood work results and physician's orders are attached.

FiO_2, fraction of inspired oxygen; HR, heart rate; RR, respiratory rate; SaO_2, blood oxygen saturation; BP, blood pressure.

Simulation Scenario Introduction

Situation/Transition	Facilitator Action	Expected Student Behavioral Outcomes	Resources
Orientation	1. Describe the setting. 2. Describe simulation experience. 3. Review simulator function (if needed).		• Simulator Directions for simulator manual

Pre-test (optional)	4. Administer pre-test:
	  a. Online quiz
	    or
	  b. Response system (i.e., I-clickers).
			• Pre-simulation quiz attached
			• I-clicker questions

Report (see instructor script)	5. Provide report by one of the following options:
	  a. Audio
	  b. Video
	  c. Script (instructor read)
	  d. Script (student read).
		1. Student will make notes based on key points of report.	• View RN to RN handoff report script
			• Smart phone download (audio and/or video)
			• Video

Start simulation	1. Select Scenario 9.0 program file: 2. Start simulation program.		• Simulator Directions for simulator manual
Phase I Introduction			
Physiologic state: HR 118 bpm (sinus tachycardia) RR 22 breaths/min SaO$_2$ 95 BP 102/64 mm Hg Temperature 37.9°C (100.2°F) FiO$_2$ 0.40 by rebreather mask. Arterial line PA catheter PAP 32/22 PAOP 6 RAP 3 CO 2.5 CI 1.9 SVR 400 LVSWI 34 RVSWI 22 PVR 250 IV normal saline solution at 125 mL/hr Foley 20 mL (last 2 hours) via Foley catheter Abdominal dressing: small amount of sanguineous drainage.	3. Progress patient situation Overview Recipe Card 9.0 4. Select "Phase II Body of Scenario" from simulation software menu within 5 minutes. *Recommended time to advance:* 9 minutes	1. Student assesses the patient, noting small sanguineous drainage on dressing and in Jackson-Pratt drains, increased temperature, tachycardia, and tachypnea. 2. Student assesses the hemodynamic lines—septic shock profile noted. 3. Student notes increased white blood count and other blood abnormalities. 4. Student calls physician to report changes, abnormal values, and assessment findings.	• Overview Recipe Card 9.0

(Continued)

Situation/Transition	Facilitator Action	Expected Student Behavioral Outcomes	Resources
Phase II Body of Scenario			
Physiologic state: HR 124 bpm sinus tachycardia with increasing PVCs. RR 24 breaths/min SaO_2 92% BP 86/46 mm Hg Temperature 38.4°C FiO_2 0.70 by rebreather mask Arterial line PA catheter IV normal saline solution at 125 mL/hr 1 liter normal saline bolus administered Foley 20 cc (last 2 hours) via Foley catheter Abdominal dressing and Jackson-Pratt drains same as earlier. Patient becomes increasingly short of breath with decreasing level of consciousness and decreasing blood pressure. ABGs pH 7.29 pCO_2 33 HCO_3 18 pO_2 78	5. Progress patient's situation following Overview Recipe Card 9.0 6. Select "Phase II Conclusion" from simulation software menu within 10 minutes. *Recommended time to advance:* 10 minutes	1. Student identifies patient's worsening condition and administers fluid boluses of normal saline as ordered. 2. Student is able to discuss hemodynamic profile of septic shock and expected management. 3. Student can accurately calculate IV drip rate for vasoactive agents as ordered and titrate agents according to the patient's response and predetermined parameters. 4. Student accurately interprets ABG values (metabolic acidosis, partially compensated, mild hypoxemia) 5. Student notifies physician immediately of change in the patient's status. 6. Student implements sepsis orders.	• Overview Recipe Card 9.0
Phase III Conclusion			
Physiologic state: HR 126 bpm sinus tachycardia with increasing PVCs. RR 30 breaths/min SaO_2 90% BP 80/46 mm Hg Temperature 38.7°C FiO_2 rebreather 0.60 Arterial line PA catheter IV normal saline solution at 125 mL/hr Another 1 liter bolus normal saline initiated Dopamine drip initiated and titrated to 15 mcg/kg/min to attempt to increase systolic BP to 90 ABGs pH 7.28 pCO_2 22 HCO_3 16 pO_2 68		1. The student recognizes the continued deterioration in the patient and notifies physician (dysrhythmias, ABG and lab value changes, decreased BP, further decreased SaO_2, increased respiratory distress and decreased level of consciousness) 2. Student prepares equipment required for intubation and consults with respiratory therapist. 3. Student assesses lab results and identifies abnormal findings. 4. Student uses advanced communication skills in an emergency situation with the patient, the family (if in attendance), and other health care team members.	• Simulator Directions for simulator manual

(Continued)

Situation/Transition	Facilitator Action	Expected Student Behavioral Outcomes	Resources
Foley 20 cc (last 2 hours) via Foley catheter Abdominal dressing and Jackson-Pratt drains same as earlier. Patient continues to deteriorate (decreased level of consciousness, mottled feet, further decreased urine output) The decision is made to intubate and prepare to initiate mechanical ventilation. Ventilator settings: SIMV 14 FiO$_2$ 0.50 PEEP 5 Neuromuscular blockade is planned BP 90/58 once dopamine titrated to 15 mcg/kg/min O$_2$ sat increases to 94 once sedated and ventilated. HR sinus tachycardia 110 bpm End simulation	7. End scenario. 8. Save debrief log.	5. Student assists physician with intubation and initiation of mechanical ventilation. 6. Sedation administered as per physician's orders. 7. Student demonstrates ability to provide a concise, thorough, hand-off report for the oncoming shift.	• Simulator Directions for simulator manual

PAP, pulmonary artery pressure; PAOP, pulmonary artery occlusive pressure; RAP, right atrial pressure; CO, cardiac output; CI, cardiac index; SVR, systemic vascular resistance; PVC, premature ventricular contraction; ABGs, arterial blood gases; SIMV, synchronized intermittent mandatory ventilation; PEEP, positive end-expiratory pressure; LWVSI, left ventricular stroke work index; RVSWI, right ventricular stroke work index; PVR, pulmonary vascular resistance.

Simulation Follow-up

Situation/Transition	Instructor Action	Expected Student Behavioral Outcomes	Resources

Debriefing	1. Allow students to discuss experience.
	2. Discuss student performance.
	3. Watch video of simulation (optional).
	4. Administer post-test:
	  a. Online quiz.
	  b. Response system.
	5. Administer post-simulation survey (optional).
	6. Instruct students to complete self-evaluation/reflection (optional).
	7. Provide remediation, if needed.
		1. Student demonstrates ability to reflect on the scenario and discusses actions that were appropriate and interventions to modify for next time.
		2. Student completes post-test.
			• Debriefing/Reflection guide
			• Post-simulation quiz
			• I-clicker questions
			Morton, P., & Fontaine, D. (2009). In *Critical care nursing: A holistic approach* (9th ed., Chapter 13). Philadelphia: Lippincott Williams & Wilkins.
			• Simulation Student Workbook septic shock follow-up questions.

Lab Results

Patient Identification
John French
Unique number: 1786811

Test	Result	Normal Ranges
Chemistry Panel:		
Sodium	130	135–1425mEq/L
Chloride	101	98–107 mEq/L
Potassium	4.1	3.5–5.1 mEq/L
Magnesium		1.3–2.1 mEq/L
BUN	5.0	6–20 mg/dL
		(Elderly >60 years old: 8–23 mg/dL)
Creatinine	100	0.4–1.3 mg/dL
Carbon dioxide, _____ total		22–30 mEq/L
Glucose	85	62–110 mg/dL
Lactate	35	5–20 mg/dL
Calcium		8.6–10.3 mg/dL
Ionized calcium		4.8–5.2
Phosphorus		2.4–5.1
HbA1C		4.0–6.7% (of total hemoglobin H)
BNP		<100 pg/mL (or <100 ng/L)
CBC:		
WBC	16.1	4.5–11.0 × 10^3
RBC	4.46	Men: 4.6–6.2 × 10^6
		Women: 4.2–5.4 × 10^6
Hgb	148	Men: 14.0–17.4 g/dL
		Women: 12.0–16. 0 g/dL
Hct	38	Men: 42–52%
		Women: 37–47%
Platelets	140	150–300 × 10^3

Test	Result	Normal Ranges
PT		12–14 seconds
PTT		18–28 seconds
INR		0.8–1.2
ALT	14	7–56 U/L
ALP	45	38–126 U/L
Amylase		30–110 U/L
AST	30	<35u/L
Ammonia		15–45 mcg/dL
Troponin I		<0.03 ng/mL
Cortisol	33	5–23 mcg/dL
Urine specific gravity	1.040	1.005–1.030
Arterial Blood Gases:		
Blood pH	7.34	7.34–7.44
HCO_3	24	22–26 mEq/L
pCO_2	49	35–45 mm Hg
pO_2	80	75–100

BUN, blood urea nitrogen; HbA1C, hemoglobin A1C; CBC, complete blood count; WBC, white blood cell; Hgb, hemoglobin; Hct, hematocrit; PT, prothrombin time; PTT, partial thromboplastin time; INR, international normalized ratio; ALT, alanine transaminase; ALP, alkaline phosphatase; AST, aspartate aminotransferase, HCO_3, bicarbonate.

Simulation Hospital

Physician's Order Record

John French
Unique Patient Number: 1786805
Hospital File

1. Use ballpoint pen.
2. Draw a line through orders not required and initial.

Admitting diagnosis: Bowel perforation and resection Allergies: No known drug allergies	Code Status: Full

Monitoring:
- ✓ Record VS q5min until stable then q1h
- ✓ Continuous cardiac monitoring
- ✓ CVP q1h
- ✓ Pulmonary capillary occlusive pressure q2h
- ✓ Cardiac output/cardiac index/SVR q_____ 4_____ h

Activity:
- ✓ Bed rest
- ✓ Position patient supine with HOB raised_____ degrees
*keep HOB raised >30 degrees when possible

Diet:
- ✓ NPO
- ☐ Heart smart
- ☐ 1800 kcal diabetic diet
- ☐ Enteral feedings: Insert small-bore feeding tube and commence feeding.
Type _____ Rate _____
- ✓ Consult dietitian

IV:
Total fluid to infuse _____ hourly
- ✓ NS at 125 mL/hr through side port
- ☐ Lactated Ringer's at _____ /hr
- ☐ NS at 50 mL/hr via RAP
- ☐ Other:_____
- ✓ Hemodynamic lines to maintain patency with NS under pressure

O_2:
Titrate O_2 to maintain SaO_2 >95%
If mechanically ventilated:
ETT inserted by _____ at _____ cm

Mode:
_____ SIMV_____ Assist Control _____ Pressure Support _____ Pressure
Control _____ CPAP
Rate:_____ Tidal volume _____
FiO_2 _____ PEEP_____
- ☐ Withhold sedation at 0600 for assessment of weaning

(Continued)

Medications:
- ☐ Aspirin, enteric coated_____ mg PO daily
- ☐ Acetaminophen 650 mg PO q6h PRN for pain or temperature >38.5° C
- ✓ Ceftazidime 500 mg IV q8h
- ☐ Cefazolin 1g IV q8h
- ☐ Dalteparin 5000 units SQ daily
- ☐ Furosemide_____ mg IV daily
- ☐ Fentanyl_____ mcg q1h PRN
- ✓ Heparin 5000 units SQ q12h
- ☐ Hydromorphone 0.5–1.0 mg IV q1h PRN
- ☐ Metoprolol_____ PO/ng_____
- ☐ Midazolam 2–4 mg IV q1–2h PRN
- ☐ Morphine_____ IV q1–2h PRN
- ☐ Ondansetron 4 mg q_____ h PRN
- ☐ Insulin Protocol

capillary blood glucose q2h

Goal 80 to 110 mg/dL

Blood glucose = Units/hour

Less than 70 = off

70–89 = 0.2 unit/hour

90–99 = 0.5 unit/hour

100–129 = 1 unit/hour

130–179= 1.5 unit/hour

180–239 = 2 unit/hour

240–299 = 3 unit/hour

300–359 = 4 unit/hour

20 notify physician
- ☐ Vancomycin _____ g q _____ h IV

Infusions:
- ☐ Voluven _____ mL if urine output <0.5 mL/kg/hr or CVP less than _____
- ☐ Nitroglycerin 100 mg/250 mL D_5W at _____ mcg/hr to maximum _____ . Titrate for chest pain
- ✓ Dopamine 400 mg/250 mL D_5W start at 5 mcg/kg/min titrate to maintain systolic BP >90.
- ☐ Epinephrine 2 mg/250 mL NS at _____ to _____ mcg/min to maintain _____ greater than _____
- ☐ Dobutamine 250 mg/250 mL NS or D_5W at _____ to_____ to maintain _____ greater than _____
- ☐ Norepinephrine 4 mg/250 mL D_5W at _____ to_____ maintain _____
- ☐ Vasopressin 20 units/hr_____ to_____to maintain _____ greater than _____
- ✓ Other: hydrocortisone 100 mg IV q6h

Chest pain protocol:

If chest pain occurs, obtain stat ECG.
- ☐ Nitroglycerin 0.4 mg spray SL PRN for chest pain. May repeat q5min × 2 (maximum 3 doses). Then notify physician

12-lead ECG on arrival
- ✓ Repeat ECG daily

Lab tests:
- ☐ Albumin daily
- ☐ Bilirubin daily
- ✓ CBC daily
- ✓ Chemistry daily (electrolytes, glucose, urea, creatinine)
- ☐ Cardiac enzymes and troponin q8h × 3
- ☐ Cross and type_____ units
- ✓ ABG daily and PRN

(Continued)

☐ Calcium daily ☐ Magnesium daily ☐ PTT/PT daily ✓ If patient becomes febrile, obtain blood for culture × 2.	
Diagnostic tests: ✓ Chest x-ray (portable) daily ☐ Echo ☐ Ultrasound_____ ☐ CT scan_____	
Treatments: ☐ Daily weights ✓ Delirium score BID ✓ Change dressing as per protocol ☐ Physiotherapy	
Other:	

Physician's Signature:_____ Date_____ Time_____
Nurse's Signature:_____ Date_____ Time_____

Pre- and Post-test Questions

Pre-test Questions	Expected Answer/Reference
1. What presenting signs and symptoms would you expect of someone in septic shock?	Altered level of consciousness, tachypnea, tachycardia, SaO_2 <90%, PaO_2 <70 mm Hg, hypotension, oliguria or anuria, fever, and increased WBC count. Dennison, R. (2007). *Pass CCRN!* (p. 707). St. Louis: Mosby. Morton, P., & Fontaine, D. (2009). *Critical care nursing: A holistic approach* (9th ed., p. 1392). Philadelphia: Lippincott Williams & Wilkins.
2. What hemodynamic profile would a patient in septic shock likely present with?	Early septic shock hemodynamic profile typically includes decreased SVR, RAP, PAP, PAOP and increased CO, CI, I, SvO_2 Dennison, R. (2007). *Pass CCRN!* (p. 84). St. Louis: Mosby.
3. Severe sepsis has a mortality rate of _____ ?	Severe sepsis has a mortality rate ranging between 40% and 70%. Morton, P., & Fontaine, D. (2009). *Critical care nursing: A holistic approach* (9th ed., p. 1391). Philadelphia: Lippincott Williams & Wilkins.

Post-test Questions	Expected Answer/Reference
1. What laboratory and diagnostic studies are helpful in diagnosing septic shock?	Lab and diagnostic tests helpful in determining septic shock include • Cultures (blood, sputum, urine, surgical or nonsurgical wounds, invasive lines) • CBC (WBC is usually elevated) • ABGs metabolic acidosis and mild hypoxemia with possible respiratory alkalosis as a compensatory mechanism. • CT scan to identify potential abscesses. • SvO_2 levels • Lactate level • $EtCO_2$ to assess for global tissue perfusion issues. Morton, P., & Fontaine, D. (2009). *Critical care nursing: A holistic approach* (9th ed., p. 1395) Philadelphia: Lippincott Williams & Wilkins.
2. What "red flag" signs or indications that your patient's condition was worsening did you observe in the simulation scenario?	Serum lactate levels and WBC increasing Increased respiratory distress and crackles in lung bases Increasing heart rate with PVCs Morton, P., & Fontaine, D. (2009). *Critical care nursing: A holistic approach* (9th ed., p. 1395) Philadelphia: Lippincott Williams & Wilkins.
3. Why are inotropes and vasopressors used as therapy in septic shock? What are the common vasoactive IV agents used in septic shock?	When fluid therapy is no longer effective, vasoactive agents should be administered to improve tissue perfusion and normalize cellular metabolism. Examples of vasoactive IV agents used for this purpose include dopamine, epinephrine, phenylephrine, dobutamine, norepinephrine, and vasopressin. These agents are titrated according to patient's response and constantly reevaluated. Surviving Sepsis Campaign: International Guidelines for management of sepsis and severe septic shock. *Intensive Care Medicine,* 36(1), 296–327.

SvO_2, tissue oxygenation; ABGs, arterial blood gases; CT, computed tomography; $EtCO_2$, end tidal carbon dioxide.

Competency Checklist

Septic Shock Case 9.0

Name: **Date:**

Competency	Examples	Met	Unmet	Comments
Performs appropriate assessment.	Comprehensive			
12- and 15-lead ECG proficiency.	Performs 12-lead ECG 12-lead ECG interpretation Performs 15-lead ECG			
Demonstrates ability to correctly interpret arrhythmia.	• Sinus rhythm with PVCs • Sinus tachycardia			
Demonstrates safe management of hemodynamic monitoring.	Pulmonary artery catheter CVP/CO/PAOP Hemodynamic profile analysis Arterial catheter			
Demonstrates safe management of oxygenation.	Ventilation modes Arterial blood gas interpretation Troubleshoots ventilator alarms			
Demonstrates safe administration of pharmacological agents.	Morphine Dopamine infusion Fluid boluses Cefazidime			
Accurately interprets lab values.	Chemistry Hematology Arterial blood gases			
Demonstrates ability to quickly recognize and prioritize a patient's rapidly deteriorating condition.	Hypotension Decreased level of consciousness Assessment of respiratory distress Notes sanguineous drainage on abdominal dressing			
Demonstrates principles related to safe patient care.	Alarms on Accurate hand-off report Communication with patient and health care team Lines secured Independent double-checks Positioning			
Specific:	Communication with family/family conference Able to suggest anticipated ventilator changes based on ABGs and changing patient's condition Suctions ETT as appropriate Follows best practice guidelines for VAP prevention			

Feedback:_____

_____

_____

_____

_____

Instructor:_____

Drug Overdose Case 10.0

Overview Recipe Card

Patient: Emily Violet Jackson

Scenario 10.0

Learning objectives	The student will
	1. Perform a focused assessment based on the patient's complaint or change in the patient's status.
	2. Recognize normal and abnormal assessment findings.
	3. Prioritize interventions based on findings and assessments.
	4. Document assessment findings.
	5. Demonstrate ability to perform and systematically interpret 12-lead ECG findings.
	6. Demonstrate ability to analyze dysrhythmias and intervene appropriately.
	7. Administer medications accurately and identify indications, contraindications, and side effects associated with interventions.
	8. Call for assistance of team as appropriate and initiate an intervention for a seizure.
	9. Initiate primary ABC measures and safely manage a general seizure.
	10. Demonstrate ability to provide a concise, thorough, hand-off report to the oncoming shift.
Equipment needed	12-lead ECG machine, arterial line to pressurized normal saline solution setup, right peripheral IV line, capped left subclavian triple-lumen distal port, medial port for normal saline solution at 50 mL/hr, proximal port for D_5W with two ampules of sodium bicarbonate and 40 mEq potassium chloride at 100 mL/hr, a nasogastric tube, cardiac monitor, crash cart with defibrillator/pacemaker, no. 7 ETT, oxygen tubing (T-piece or corrugated oxygen tubing, ETT connector), suction, simulated medications, identification band for patient, role name tags for team members, clipboard with ICU flow sheet, lab results, 12-lead ECG results and physician's orders, telephone, and code blue button
Introduction	Administer pre-test
Body of scenario	Patient remains unresponsive since admission to the ICU after ingesting tricyclic antidepressants approximately 3 hours ago and progresses to a generalized, tonic–clonic seizure lasting <1 minute.
Conclusion	Patient stabilizes after receiving a pharmacological intervention as evidenced by reaction to noxious/painful stimuli.
Debriefing	Administer post-test

ETT, endotracheal tube.

Critical Care Simulation

Drug Overdose Case 10.0

<table>
<tr>
<td>

Scenario number: 10.0
Scenario focus: Drug overdose (tricyclic antidepressants)
Scenario level: Critical care
Admission type: ICU
Patient name: Emily Violet Jackson
Unique number: 1786609
Case number: 10.0
Date of birth: December 18, 1993
Age: 18
Gender: F
Attending: Karl Busch, MD
Scenario start day: Friday
Scenario start time: 1100
Admitting diagnosis: Drug overdose
Primary diagnosis: Ingestion tricyclic antidepressants
Secondary diagnosis: Major depressive disorder
Recommended scenario time limit: 20–25 minutes
Recommended debriefing time limit: 20–30 minutes

</td>
<td>

Scenario purpose: Nursing management of a patient experiencing a drug overdose (tricyclic antidepressants) and subsequent seizure in a critical care practice setting.

Learning objectives:
The student will
1. Perform a focused assessment based on the patient's complaint or change in the patient's status.
2. Recognize normal and abnormal assessment findings.
3. Prioritize interventions based on findings and assessments.
4. Document assessment findings.
5. Demonstrate ability to perform and systematically interpret 12-lead ECG findings.
6. Demonstrate ability to analyze dysrhythmias and intervene appropriately.
7. Administer medications accurately and identify indications, contraindications, and side effects associated with interventions.
8. Call for assistance of team as appropriate and initiate an intervention for a seizure.
9. Initiate primary ABC measures and safely manage a general seizure.
10. Demonstrate ability to provide a concise, thorough, hand-off report to the oncoming shift.

Learning resources:
Reading assignment:
Bickley, L., & Szilagyi, P. (2009). *Bates' guide to physical examination and history taking* (10th ed.). Philadelphia: Lippincott Williams & Wilkins.
Diepenbrock, N. (2012). *Quick reference to critical care* (4th ed.). Philadelphia: Lippincott Williams & Wilkins.
ICU/ER Facts Made Incredibly Easy. (2011). Philadelphia: Lippincott Williams & Wilkins. *Will be added when published*
Karch, A. (2011). *Nursing drug guide.* Philadelphia: Lippincott Williams & Wilkins.
Morton, P., & Fontaine, D. (2009). *Critical care nursing: A holistic approach* (9th ed.). Philadelphia: Lippincott, Williams & Wilkins.
Simulation Student Workbook activities: Drug overdose 10.0 in student workbook. Student to complete pre-simulation.

</td>
</tr>
</table>

RN to RN Handoff Report

Emily Jackson is an 18-year-old female patient of Dr. Busch. She was admitted from the ER with a tricyclic antidepressant overdose. A university student in her first year, it was reported that Emily was becoming more despondent over the past 6–8 weeks. She lives in the university residence, where her roommate noted her having difficulty in sleeping, becoming apprehensive, and not eating well. Approximately 2 weeks ago she stopped going to the cafeteria for her meals. Before admission to hospital 3 hours ago, Emily's roommate found her on the sofa; she was unresponsive and had dry flushed skin and a pool of vomit around her head. Paramedics found an empty vial of her roommate's medication for amitriptyline. It is estimated that the vial contained amitriptyline 10 mg tablets, with approximately 90 tablets remaining. It had been over 3 hours since someone had spoken to Emily. The paramedics intubated her with a no. 7 endotracheal tube to protect the airway, administered oxygen via a T-piece, and established a large-bore right antecubital peripheral IV line. They also inserted a right radial arterial line; a left subclavian triple-lumen catheter (distal port is capped, medial port infusing normal saline solution at 50 mL/hr, proximal port infusing D_5W with two ampules of sodium bicarbonate and 40 mEq potassium chloride at 100 mL/hr); she has a nasogastric tube via the left nare and a no. 16 Foley catheter. A call was placed to Poison Control which recommended administering activated charcoal 50 g with sorbitol via nasogastric tube stat and repeated q6h twice.

Blood pressure 98/60 mm Hg, heart rate 120 bpm, respiratory rate 12 bpm, SaO_2 95%, urine output in the last hour is 100 mL, pale-yellow urine.

Patient has environmental allergies.

Past history: tonsillectomy, age 6

Blood work results and physician's orders are attached.

Simulation Scenario

Situation/Transition	Facilitator Action	Expected Student Behavioral Outcomes	Resources
Orientation	1. Describe the setting 2. Describe simulation experience 3. Review simulator function (if needed)		• Simulator Directions for simulator manual

Pre-test (optional)	4. Administer pre-test:
	  a. Online quiz
	    or
	  b. Response system (i.e., I-clickers)
			• Pre-simulation quiz attached
			• I-clicker questions

Report (see instructor script)	5. Provide report by one of the following options:
	  a. Audio
	  b. Video
	  c. Script (instructor read)
	  d. Script (student read).
		1. Student will make notes based on key points of report.	• View RN to RN Handoff Report
			• Smart phone download (audio and/or video)
			• Video

Start simulation	1. Select Scenario 10.0 program file 2. Start simulation program. Set up vital signs and beginning of patient parameters.		• Simulator Directions for simulator manual
Phase I Introduction			
Physiologic state: HR 120 bpm (sinus rhythm with widened QRS complex 0.16) BP 98/60 mm Hg via right radial arterial line RR 12 breaths/min SaO₂ 95% on FiO₂ 0.35 via T-piece Temperature 35.1°C Urinary output 150 mL, pale-yellow urine Pupils: 4 mm, react briskly to light	1. Progress patient situation following Overview Recipe Card 10.0 *Recommended time to advance scenario:* 10 minutes	1. Student conducts systematic patient assessment. 2. Student checks orders and lab values and calculates IV drip rates for accuracy. Student also verbalizes understanding of medications, indications, and side effects parameters to assess. 3. Student assesses all hemodynamic lines, waveforms, and values and demonstrates correct method for zeroing, leveling and calibrating equipment. 4. Student compares cuff blood pressure to intra-arterial pressure. 5. Student analyzes cardiac rhythm accurately. 6. Student uses advanced communication strategies when communicating with the patient, the patient's family, and other members of the health care team. 7. Student documents accurately on ICU flow sheet.	• Overview Recipe Card 10.0

(Continued)

Situation/Transition	Facilitator Action	Expected Student Behavioral Outcomes	Resources
		8. Student notes sinus tachycardia with widened QRS complex and asks to see and interpret 12-lead ECG accurately. 9. Student demonstrates ability to accurately interpret blood work and recognizes abnormal values. 10. Student demonstrates ability to manage an intubated patient spontaneously breathing via T-piece.	
Phase II Body of Scenario			
Physiologic state: Patient begins to have a tonic–clonic seizure; arms and legs stiffen and extend, apnea, skin color is pale and dusky, seizure lasts approximately 20 seconds. Then the patient has rhythmic muscle contractions, the patient hyperventilates, followed by diaphoresis and tachycardia lasting 30 seconds. Then the patient becomes flaccid. HR 140 bpm (sinus rhythm with widened QRS complex 0.16) BP 110/60 mm Hg via right radial arterial line RR 24 breaths/min SaO_2 92% on FiO_2 0.35 via T-piece Temperature 35.1°C Urinary output 150 mL, pale-yellow urine Pupils: 4 mm and left reacts briskly to light, while right reacts sluggishly	3. Progress patient situation following Overview Recipe Card 10.0 4. Select "Phase II Outcome" from simulation software menu within 10 minutes *Recommended time to advance scenario:* 5 minutes Provides 12-lead ECG Provide Stat Lab Results #2	1. Student demonstrates ability to recognize tonic–clonic seizure and protects patient during seizure. Student calls for assistance of colleagues and directs colleagues to administer lorazepam (Ativan) 2 mg IV push. 2. Student performs a focused neurological assessment after seizure activity ceases. 3. Student sends blood to lab for electrolyte, AGB, and glucose analysis. 4. Student asks for ECG and accurately interprets it. 5. Student accurately interprets lab results.	• Overview Recipe Card 10.0
Phase III Conclusion of Scenario			
Physiologic state: HR 110 bpm (sinus rhythm with widened QRS complex 0.16) BP 90/60 mm Hg via right radial arterial line RR 12 bpm SaO_2 95% on FiO_2 0.35 via T-piece Temperature 36.1°C Urinary output 150 mL, pale-yellow urine Pupils: 4 mm and react briskly to light bilaterally Reacts to noxious/painful stimuli *End simulation*		1. Student performs neurological reassessment and documents. 2. Student updates family regarding patient condition.	Prepare to go to debriefing session.

SaO_2, blood oxygen saturation; FiO_2, fraction of inspired oxygen; ABG, arterial blood gas; HR, heart rate; RR, respiratory rate.

Simulation Follow-up

Situation/Transition	Instructor Action	Expected Student Behavioral Outcomes	Resources

Debriefing	1. Allow students to discuss experience
	2. Discuss students' performance
	3. Watch video of simulation (optional)
	4. Administer post-test (attached)
	  a. Online quiz
	  b. Response system
	5. Administer post-simulation survey (optional)
	6. Instruct students to complete self-evaluation/reflection (optional)
	7. Provide remediation, if needed
		1. Student demonstrates ability to reflect on the scenario and discusses actions that were appropriate and interventions to modify for next time.
		2. Student completes post-test.
			I-clicker questions
			Post-test
			Simulation Student Workbook follow-up assignment

Lab Results

Patient Identification
Emily Violet Jackson
Unique number: 1786815

Test	Result	Normal Ranges
Chemistry Panel:		
Sodium	132	135–1425 mEq/L
Chloride	101	98–107 mEq/L
Potassium	3.5	3.5–5.1 mEq/L
Magnesium	1.2	1.3–2.1 mEq/L
BUN	8.3	6–20 mg/dL (Elderly >60 years old: 8–23 mg/dL)
Creatinine	1.2	0.4–1.3 mg/dL
Carbon dioxide, total		22–30 mEq/L
Glucose	68	62–110 mg/dL
Lactate		5–20 mg/dL
Calcium		8.6–10.3 mg/dL
Ionized calcium		4.8–5.2
Phosphorus		2.4–5.1
HbA1C		4.0%–6.7% (of total hemoglobin H)
BNP		<100 pg/mL (or <100 ng/L)
CBC:		
WBC	12.1	$4.5–11.0 \times 10^3$
RBC	4.46	Men: $4.6–6.2 \times 10^6$ Women: $4.2–5.4 \times 10^6$
Hgb	13.8	Men: 14.0–17.4 g/dL Women: 12.0–16.0 g/dL
Hct	41	Men: 42–52% Women: 37–47%
Platelets		$150–300 \times 10^3$

BUN, blood urea nitrogen; CBC, complete blood count; WBC, white blood cells; RBC, red blood cells; Hgb, hemoglobin.

Test	Result	Normal Ranges
PT **PTT** **INR**		12–14 seconds 18–28 seconds 0.8–1.2
Liver Enzymes: ALT ALP Amylase Troponin I Serum lactate: <u>Arterial Blood Gases:</u> Blood pH HCO_3 pCO_2 pO_2	12 42 7.33 15 25 85	7–56 U/L 38–126 U/L 30–110 U/L <0.03 ng/mL 5–20 mg/dL 7.34–7.44 22–26 mEq/L 35–45 mm Hg 75–100

PT, prothrombin time; PTT, partial thromboplastin time; INR, international normalized ratio; ALT, alanine transaminase; ALP, alkaline phosphatase.

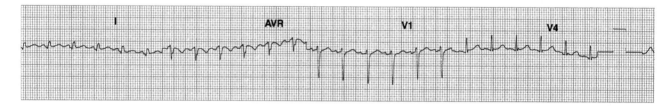

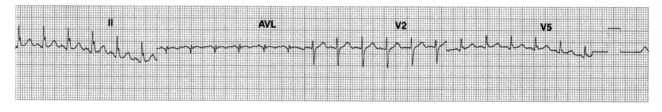

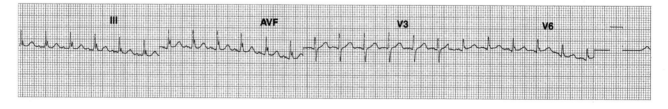

Stat Lab Results

Date/Time:_____ Patient Name: <u>Emily Jackson</u>
Unique Patient Number: 1786815

Hematology Hgb:_____Hct:_____ WBC:_____ Platelets:_____ Other	Chemistry Na: <u>132</u> K: <u>3.9</u> Cl: <u>110</u> HCO$_3$: <u>17</u> Urea: <u>7</u> Creatinine: ˙<u>100</u> Glucose: <u>5</u> CPK: _____Troponin: _____ AST: _____ALT: _____ Other: ABGs: pH 7.32, PCO$_2$ 25, PO$_2$ 80, HCO$_3$ 18
Coagulation studies PT:_____ PTT:_____ INR:_____ Bleeding time:_____ D-dimers:_____ Fibrin split products:_____ Other	Urinalysis pH:_____ Glucose:_____ Ketones:_____ Specific gravity:_____ Blood:_____ Protein:_____ Leukocytes:_____

Emily Violet Jackson.

Simulation Hospital

Physician's Order Record

Emily Violet Jackson
Unique Patient Number: 1786815

1. Use ballpoint pen.
2. Draw a line through orders not required and initial your changes.

Admitting diagnosis: Drug overdose tricyclic antidepressants, major depressive disorder Allergies: Environmental	Code status: Full

Monitoring:
    ✓   Record VS q15min until stable then q1h
    ✓   Continuous cardiac monitoring
    ☐   CVP q1h
    ☐   Pulmonary artery occlusive pressure q_h
    ☐ Cardiac output/cardiac index/SVR q_h	

Activity:
    ✓   Bed rest
    ☐   Position supine with HOB raised _____degrees
*Keep HOB raised more than 30 degrees when possible	

(Continued)

Diet:
- ✓ NPO
- ☐ Heart smart
- ☐ 1800 kcal diabetic diet
- ☐ Enteral feedings: Insert small-bore feeding tube and commence feeding.

Type _____ Rate _____
- ✓ Consult dietitian

IV:

Total fluid to infuse 150 mL/hr
- ✓ NS at 50 mL/hr
- ☐ Lactated Ringer's solution at _____/hr
- ✓ D$_5$W at 100 mL/hr
- ☐ Other: Two ampules of sodium bicarbonate per liter and 40 mEq KCl
- ✓ Hemodynamic lines to maintain patency with NS under pressure

O$_2$:

Titrate O$_2$ to maintain SaO$_2$ at more than 94%

If mechanically ventilated:

ETT inserted by RT at 22 cm

Place on T-piece FiO$_2$ 0.35

Mode:

_____ SIMV _____ Assist Control _____ Pressure Support _____ Pressure Control _____ CPAP

Rate:_____ Tidal volume_____

FiO$_2$_____ PEEP_____
- ☐ Withhold sedation at 0600 for assessment of weaning

Medications:
- ☐ Aspirin enteric coated _____ mg PO daily
- ✓ Acetaminophen 650 mg PO q6h PRN pain or temperature more than 38.5°C
- ☐ Ceftazidime 500 mg IV q8h
- ☐ Cefazolin 1 g IV q8h
- ☐ Dalteparin 5000 units SQ daily
- ☐ Furosemide _____ mg IV daily
- ☐ Fentanyl _____ mcg q1h PRN
- ☐ Heparin 5000 units SQ q12h
- ☐ Hydromorphone 0.5–1.0 mg IV q1h PRN
- ☐ Metoprolol _____ PO/ng _____
- ☐ Midazolam 2–4 mg IV q1–2h PRN
- ☐ Morphine _____ IV q1–2h PRN
- ☐ Ondansetron 4 mg q _____ h PRN
- ☐ Insulin Protocol

capillary blood glucose q2h

Goal 80 to 110 mg/dL

Blood glucose = Units/hour

Less than 70 = off

70–89 = 0.2 unit/hour

90–99 = 0.5 unit/hour

100–129 = 1 unit/hour

130–179 = 1.5 unit/hour

180–239 = 2 unit/hour

240–299 = 3 unit/hour

300–359 = 4 unit/hour

20 notify physician
- ☐ Vancomycin _____ g q _____ h IV

(Continued)

Infusions:

- ✓ Voluven _____mL if urine output <0.5 mL/kg/hr or CVP <_____
- ☐ Nitroglycerin 100 mg/250 mL D$_5$W at _____mcg/hr to max_____. Titrate for chest pain
- ✓ Dopamine 200 mg/250 mL D$_5$W at <u>3 mcg/kg/min to 15 mcg/kg</u>/min titrate to maintain systolic blood pressure >$\underline{100}$ mm Hg
- ☐ Epinephrine 2 mg/250 mL NS at _____to _____mcg/min to maintain _____>_____
- ☐ Dobutamine 250 mg/250 mL NS or D$_5$W at_____to _____to maintain _____>_____
- ☐ Norepinephrine 4 mg/250 mL D$_5$W at_____to _____maintain _____
- ☐ Vasopressin 20 U/hr _____to _____to maintain _____>_____
- ☐ Other

Chest pain protocol:

If chest pain occurs, obtain stat ECG,

- ☐ Nitroglycerin 0.4 mg spray SL PRN for chest pain. May repeat q5min × 2 (maximum 3 doses). Then notify physician.

12-lead ECG on arrival

- ✓ Repeat ECG q8h

Lab tests:

- ☐ Albumin daily
- ☐ Bilirubin daily
- ✓ CBC daily
- ✓ Chemistry daily (electrolytes, glucose, urea, creatinine)
- ☐ Cardiac enzymes and troponin q8h × 3
- ☐ Cross and type _____units
- ✓ ABG daily and PRN
- ✓ Calcium daily
- ✓ Magnesium daily
- ✓ PTT/PT daily
- ✓ If patient becomes febrile, obtain blood for culture × 2

Diagnostic tests:

- ✓ Chest x-ray (portable) daily
- ☐ Echo
- ☐ Ultrasound_____
- ☐ CT scan_____

Treatments:

- ☐ Daily weights
- ✓ Delirium score twice daily
- ☐ Change dressing as per protocol
- ✓ Physiotherapy

Other:

Activated charcoal 50 g with sorbitol q4h × 2

lorazepam (Ativan) 2–4 mg for seizures PRN

Monitor telemetry for widening of the QRS

Physician's Signature:_____ Date:_____ Time:_____
Nurse's Signature:_____ Date:_____ Time:_____

Pre- and Post-Test Questions

Pre-test Questions	Expected Answer/Reference
1. List the antidotes for acetaminophen, anticholinergics, benzodiazepines, cyclic antidepressants, digoxin, heparin, opiates, and warfarin	Acetaminophen: N-acetylcysteine Anticholinergics: Physostigmine Benzodiazepines: Flumazenil Cyclic antidepressants, sodium bicarbonate Digoxin: Digoxin immune fab Heparin: Protamine sulfate Opiates: Naloxone Warfarin: Vitamin K Karch, A. (2011). *Nursing drug guide*. Philadelphia: Lippincott Williams & Wilkins. Morton, P., & Fontaine, D. (2009). *Critical care nursing: A holistic approach* (9th ed., p. 1444). Philadelphia: Lippincott Williams & Wilkins.
2. Describe the signs and symptoms of a TCA overdose.	Signs and symptoms of a TCA overdose: hypotension, tachycardia, supraventricular tachycardia, ventricular dysrhythmias, conduction defects, myocardial infarction, cardiopulmonary arrest, seizures, CNS depression, metabolic acidosis Morton, P., & Fontaine, D. (2009). *Critical care nursing: A holistic approach* (9th ed., p. 1449). Philadelphia: Lippincott Williams & Wilkins.
3. Why is it important to alkalinize the blood of a patient experiencing a TCA overdose?	Alkalinizing the blood may control ventricular dysrhythmias and improve conduction delays by keeping the pH 7.45–7.55. This may be done by bolus doses of sodium bicarbonate or through intubation and ventilation. Morton, P., & Fontaine, D. (2009). *Critical care nursing: A holistic approach* (9th ed., p. 1440). Philadelphia: Lippincott Williams & Wilkins.

TCA, tricyclic antidepressant; CNS, central nervous system.

Post-test Questions	Expected Answer/Reference
1. Discuss nursing management for a patient experiencing a seizure.	• Protect the patient from injury: Raise and pad side rails, keep suction and oral airway at bedside, position patient in lateral recumbent position, provide suction to prevent aspiration, assess neurovital signs • Observe for complications • Administer pharmacological interventions Hickey, J. (2009). *The clinical practice of neurological & neurosurgical nursing* (6th ed., p. 658). Philadelphia: Lippincott Williams & Wilkins.
2. Describe key priorities when managing a patient experiencing a drug overdose, such as tricyclic overdose.	Airway: Maintain patent airway, position patient to prevent aspiration, intubate and ventilate patient • Breathing: Ventilate to manage respiratory depression as well as to manipulate ABG values • Circulation: Maintain adequate circulating volume with IV fluids, dopamine, or norepinephrine bitartrate (Levophed) infusions • Seizures: Ensure environmental safety, prepare for pharmacological interventions with IV benzodiazepines and an anticonvulsant • Lab results: Screen electrolytes, ABG values, glucose, creatinine, complete blood count, urinalysis, and toxicology results • Health promotion: If unintentional overdose, discuss with patient medication reconciliation, and consult pharmacist • Suicide attempt: Provide counseling and referral Morton, P., & Fontaine, D. (2009). *Critical care nursing: A holistic approach* (9th ed., pp. 1439–1449). Philadelphia: Lippincott Williams & Wilkins.
3. Describe the anion gap and the significance of the anion gap for patients experiencing a drug overdose.	Calculation of the anion gap is a method of evaluating the difference between measured and unmeasured cations (positively charged particles such as sodium) and measured and unmeasured anions (negatively charged particles such as bicarbonate). The formula is calculated: $[Na] - ([Cl] + [HCO_3]) =$ anion gap Normal is 8–16 mEq/L: <8 mEq/L indicates hyponatremia, hypermagnesemia, multiple myeloma, or hypoalbuminemia; >16 mEq/L indicates a metabolic acidosis from conditions, such as diabetic ketoacidosis, uremia/renal failure, lactic acidosis from sepsis, shock, bowel ischemia, salicylates, antifreeze ingestion, or isoniazid Morton, P., & Fontaine, D. (2009). *Critical care nursing: A holistic approach* (9th ed., p. 1444). Philadelphia: Lippincott Williams & Wilkins.

ABG, arterial blood gas.

Competency Checklist

Drug Overdose Case 10.0

Name: **Date:**

Competency	Examples	Met	Unmet	Comments
Performs appropriate assessment	Comprehensive Focused neurological			
Demonstrates ability to correctly interpret arrhythmia and 12-lead ECG	Sinus tachycardia Widened QRS			
Demonstrates safe management of hemodynamic monitoring	Arterial line CVP			
Demonstrates safe management of oxygenation	T-piece Endotracheal tube Mechanical ventilation Insertion of bite block			
Demonstrates safe administration of pharmacological agents	Lorazepam			
Accurately interprets lab values	Chemistry Hematology Arterial blood gases			
Demonstrates ability to quickly recognize and prioritize a patient's rapidly deteriorating condition	Seizure management Airway management			
Demonstrates principles related to safe patient care	Alarms Lines secured Independent double checks SBAR reporting			
Specific	Draws labs from arterial line Communication with family/team			

Feedback:_____
_____
_____
_____
_____
_____

Instructor:_____

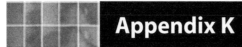
The Overview Template

Learning objectives Equipment needed Introduction Body of scenario Conclusion Debrief	The student will Administer pre-test Administer post-test

The Critical Care Simulation

Title of the Case:_____

Scenario number: **Scenario focus:** **Scenario level:** Critical care **Admission type:** ICU **Patient name:** **Unique number:** **Case number:** **Date of birth:** **Age:** **Gender:** **Attending:** **Scenario start day:** **Scenario start time:** **Admitting diagnosis:** **Primary diagnosis:** **Secondary diagnosis:** **Recommended scenario time limit:** 20–25 minutes. **Recommended debriefing time limit:** 20–30 minutes. **RN handoff report** Blood work and doctor's orders.	**Scenario purpose: Learning objectives** The student will **Learning resources:** Reading assignment: **Simulation Student Workbook activities:**

Simulation Scenario

Situation/Transition	Facilitator Action	Expected Student Behavioral Outcomes	Resources
Orientation	1. Describe the setting 2. Describe simulation experience 3. Review simulator function (if needed) 4. Assign roles and provide name tags		• Simulator Directions for simulator manual

Pre-test (optional)	5. Administer pre-test
	  a. Online quiz
	    or
	  b. Response system (i.e., I-clickers)
			• Pre-simulation quiz attached
			• I-clicker questions

Report (see instructor script)	6. Provide report by one of the following options:
	  a. Audio
	  b. Video
	  c. Script (instructor read)
	  d. Script (student read)
		1. Student will make notes based on key points of report.	• View RN-to-RN report script
			• Smart phone download (audio and/or video)
			• Video

Start simulation	1. Select scenario __ program file 2. Start simulation program		• Simulator Directions for simulator manual
Phase I Introduction			
Physiologic state:	3. Progress patient situation following Overview Recipe Card 4. Select "Phase II Experience" from simulation software menu within 10 minutes *Recommended time to advance:* 10 minutes		• Overview Recipe Card #_____
Phase II Body of Scenario			
	5. Progress patient situation following Overview Recipe Card 3.0 6. Select "Phase II Outcome" from simulation software menu within 10 minutes *Recommended time to advance:* 5–10 minutes		• Overview Recipe Card #_____
Phase III Conclusion			
End simulation	7. End scenario 8. Save debrief log		• Simulator Directions for Use manual

Simulation Follow-up

Situation/Transition	Facilitator Action	Expected Student Behavioral Outcomes	Resources
Debriefing	1. Allow students to discuss experience 2. Discuss student performance 3. Watch video of simulation (optional) 4. Administer post-test 5. Online quiz 6. Response system 7. Administer post-simulation survey (optional) 8. Instruct students to complete self-evaluation/reflection (optional) 9. Provide remediation, if needed	1. Student demonstrates ability to reflect on the scenario and discusses actions that were appropriate and interventions to modify for next time. 2. Student completes post-test	• Debriefing/reflection guide • Post-simulation quiz • Textbook readings: • Simulation Student Workbook Activities:

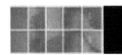

Glossary

Authenticity: how true to life the setting has been created

Environmental Fidelity: refers to the realism of the environment

Fidelity: degree of realism

Formative Evaluation: feedback after small achievements throughout the performance, builds confidence

Guided Reflection: through the use of prompting cues, reviewing performance or practice

Psychological Fidelity: the degree to which the participant feels the simulation is realistic

Simulation: the "art and science of recreating a clinical situation in an artificial setting"

Simulation Recipe Card: a systematic method for implementing simulation scenarios

Summative Evaluation: evaluation of overall performance at the end of a course often affecting academic progression, may assign a "pass" or "fail"